Punishing Violence

Despite the perception of an increase in violent crime, not all violence is criminalised and many of those who suffer assault do not go to the police. Even when violence is reported, the case may never reach the courts. Who decides whether or not violent behaviour deserves punishment and what factors determine the success or failure of criminal prosecution?

Punishing Violence examines the series of decisions – by victims, police officers, prosecutors and courts – which determine whether violent behaviour is criminalised and offenders punished. Based on their own innovative research, Antonia Cretney and Gwynn Davis draw attention to the crucial role of the victim, not only in deciding whether to report violence to the police but also in determining the police response and the ultimate success or failure of the prosecution effort. They identify a serious dislocation between the purposes of victims and the purposes of the justice system.

Providing an authoritative account of the reality of assault and of its reporting, investigation and prosecution, *Punishing Violence* will be invaluable reading not only for criminologists and students but also for all those with an interest in the workings of the justice system.

Antonia Cretney is Research Fellow and **Gwynn Davis** is Senior Research Fellow in the Law Faculty at the University of Bristol.

Punishing Violence

Antonia Cretney and Gwynn Davis

London and New York

First published 1995
by Routledge
11 New Fetter Lane, London EC4P 4EE

Simultaneously published in the USA and Canada
by Routledge
29 West 35th Street, New York, NY 10001

Typeset in Times by LaserScript, Mitcham, Surrey
Printed and bound in Great Britain by
TJ Press, Padstow, Cornwall

British Library Cataloguing in Publication Data
A catalogue record for this book is available from the British Library

Library of Congress Cataloguing in Publication Data
A catalogue record for this book has been requested

ISBN 0–415–09839–4 (hbk)
ISBN 0–415–09840–8 (pbk)

Contents

Illustrations

Preface

Interpersonal violence is a matter of abiding academic and media interest. There has of late been a perceived increase in the prevalence of violent conduct, leading to a greater public awareness of violence as a problem meriting criminal sanction. In this book we explore victims' perceptions of and reaction to violence in a variety of contexts, including the 'domestic', and thereafter we describe the *response* to violent behaviour, both within the framework of criminal prosecution and independently of it. In order to do this we employed an original research design which involved our monitoring assaults in which the victims had been referred to a major city centre hospital for medical treatment. The object was to gain access to a large group of assault victims *outside* the justice system – this being essential if we were to understand reasons why many assaults are never brought to police attention. The research methodology which we employed enabled us to investigate the relationships underlying assault, the reasons for the violence, and the factors militating against police and court involvement.

The main purpose of this book, therefore, is to provide an authoritative account of the reality of assault and of its reporting, investigation and prosecution. There already exist accounts of the principles underpinning the operation of the criminal law in cases of violence, and of court decision-making in leading cases, but there has been comparatively little on the victim's role in prosecuting violence, or indeed on the prosecution process *as seen by* the victim.

The starting-point for the research underpinning this book was the Accident and Emergency Department of Bristol Royal Infirmary. The contact which we were thus able to have with individuals who recognised themselves as victims of assault gave us a unique point of departure from which to trace cases, some of which remained private incidents, others of which eventually culminated in a criminal trial. We are very much in the debt of Professor Jon Shepherd, now of Cardiff University, then of the Department of Oral Surgery in Bristol, who gave us the idea for this method of approach, who was instrumental in setting it up and who thereafter assisted our reflections on the material thus obtained. Geoff Hughes, Senior Consultant in the Accident and Emergency Department, smoothed our path as we intruded upon a very busy environment managed by hard-pressed staff. We owe particular thanks to the reception staff of the Accident and Emergency Department who allowed us to share their work-station in the small hours of the night and who furnished us with lists of those patients whom we might approach. When we visited patients on the ward the staff there, too, were generous in the assistance they gave us.

For the next stage of the research process we were heavily dependent upon the goodwill and practical help of Avon and Somerset Constabulary. In this we were fortunate to be guided by Superintendent Alun Howells, who not only provided advice and practical assistance but made us feel welcome even when we must have placed awkward demands upon his time. Similarly, the officers whose time we took up with our interviews did everything they could to assist. We are grateful to them all.

In the Bristol magistrates and crown courts we were anonymous observers, but there too we were given every possible assistance by court staff, while those prosecuting and defence lawyers whom we approached answered our queries frankly and with good humour.

The research was funded by the ESRC, to whom we are indebted for their support.

Among our colleagues in Bristol we owe particular thanks to Chris Clarkson, Stephen Jones, Pat Hammond and Mike Drew. Chris Clarkson and Stephen Jones were closely involved in the birth of the research plan and shared in the fieldwork. In the reflective process also, their contribution was invaluable. Pat Hammond dealt patiently with the research data in its many stages of development and typed the final manuscript with her usual meticulous skill. Mike Drew created our tables and gave essential assistance with some of the statistical operations.

Finally, we are indebted to the assault victims who generously met the demands we placed upon them, allowing themselves to be interviewed at length and in depth about what at best was an unpleasant incident, at worst a traumatising catastrophe. We hope that however modest the scope of this book it may go some way towards elucidating their experience.

Chapter 1

Introduction

Violent incidents comprise but a tiny fraction of the encounters which we have with our fellow men and women. Most of us subdue our violent impulses virtually all of the time. We are effectively socialised into a non-violent culture. But it is readily apparent that this is not true of all, and it is perhaps true of very few of us *in extremis*. Interpersonal violence is for this reason a matter of abiding academic and media interest. There has of late been a perceived increase in the prevalence of violent conduct, and while there may indeed have been some increase in real terms this perhaps also reflects a greater public awareness and recognition of violence as a problem meriting criminal sanction. It is possible that we have a greater sensitivity towards violence than our forebears, and a greater reluctance to tolerate its use in public or private.[1] Two questions then follow: does this greater sensitivity encourage those on the receiving end of violence to bring their victimisation to the attention of police and courts?; and, second, what is the response of criminal justice agencies to those assaults which are brought to their notice? In this book we shall focus upon a certain type of behaviour (interpersonal violence) in order to explore the *definition* of that behaviour – first by victims, and second by the police and courts – and, thereafter, to monitor the *response* to that behaviour, either within the framework of criminal prosecution or independently of it.[2] Even as we write we read of a major teaching union opting to bring private prosecutions for assault against schoolchildren who have attacked its members;[3] of complaints by the Prison Officers' Association that serious assaults by inmates upon officers and fellow prisoners have not led to criminal proceedings;[4] and of Crown Prosecution Service reluctance to level serious charges against drunk drivers who kill.[5] Does this indicate a failure on the part of agents of the state to respond effectively to flagrant breaches of the criminal law? If so, what are the reasons for this failure?

'Assault' has a technical, legal definition as well as a lay meaning. Legally speaking it covers a number of offence categories ranging from 'common assault' (punishable with a maximum penalty of a £2,000 fine and/or six months' imprisonment) to 'wounding or causing grievous bodily harm with intent' (maximum sentence: life imprisonment).[6] In addition there are various sexual assaults, of which the most serious is rape, which again carries a maximum sentence of life imprisonment. We do not take these legal definitions as our starting point. We are concerned with any physical violation through the use of force, although we should make clear at this point that we have focused principally upon non-sexual violence. Physical integrity is in general highly valued (Ashworth 1991: 277) and the violation of that integrity, through the application of force, is profoundly unwelcome. Assault, therefore, although subject to quite complex legal definition, is something to which we all respond intuitively.

This is not to say that there are *no* problems of definition, and it is inevitable that any attempt to measure the extent of violent conduct will encounter difficulties. Nonetheless it is important to make some attempt to do this and the obvious place to start is with the official record of offences of violence against the person recorded by the police. The figures reveal a dramatic increase in the number of violent offences over the past 20 years, a trend also observed in other Western countries. Thus in 1971 there were 47,000 recorded offences of violence against the person in England and Wales; in 1990 the figure had risen to 184,700; in 1991 it was 190,300; and in 1992 it was 201,800.[7] While the method of recording may have changed somewhat, rendering the figures not precisely comparable, there is no denying that an increase of over 400 per cent in 20 years is very dramatic. The rise has been most significant in respect of the less serious violent offences (Walmsley 1986: 53), although one may also note that *robbery*, which is essentially a crime of violence (Ashworth 1991: 340) and can give rise to very serious injury, also shows a striking increase. There were in fact 20,300 robberies recorded in England and Wales in 1981; 45,300 in 1991; and 52,900 in 1992.[8] In general we can say that violent offences appear to have increased more rapidly than other crimes, and this is reflected in the fact that violent offenders form an increasing proportion of the prison population.[9] The official statistics also reveal an apparently higher prosecution rate for assaults than for most other offences. Some 75 per cent of recorded violent crime is said to be cleared up – referred to by one Home Office Minister as 'a very high detection rate indeed'.[10]

It is acknowledged, not least by those responsible for gathering the figures, that criminal statistics contain many distortions. Increases in recorded crime probably reflect changes in reporting and recording practices at least as much as they do changes in the underlying crime rate. Taking first the willingness of victims (and others) to bring offences to police attention, it is probable that offences against the person, such as wounding, are among the least well reported.[11] Even victims who do report an assault may do so reluctantly (Shapland *et al.* 1985: 16), making it less likely that the offence will be recorded or an investigation pursued. Our own contact with victims living in conditions of severe deprivation (for which see Chapter 2) suggested a high level of unreported violence. Heavy drinkers, especially, may become involved in an altercation and perhaps collapse in the street, unaware that they might lay claim to being an assault victim and certainly with no intention of reporting the incident to the police.[12] As a corollary, it is possible that the recent rise in the number of woundings and other assaults reflects a greater willingness to report violence, at least in certain contexts. Most obviously there has been a marked increase in the number of 'domestic' assaults reported to the police: this almost certainly reflects a growing perception on the part of women that assaults in the home can and should be brought to police attention.[13]

The other difficulty in calculating the true level of assault arises from variations in police recording practices in respect of those incidents which are brought to their attention. There is evidence of significant non-recording (or 'cuffing', in police argot) of some categories of assault, notably those in which the police anticipate difficulty in prosecuting. One survey found that nearly a quarter of assault and wounding cases were written off (for statistical purposes) by the police, usually because the complainant did not wish the offence to be prosecuted (Sparks *et al.* 1977: 145). Those researchers observed that cases written off in this manner 'were almost invariably family disputes'. Another survey, this time of assault victims who sought hospital treatment, revealed that only one-quarter of these assaults were recorded by police although half the victims interviewed claimed police awareness of the incident (Shepherd *et al.* 1989). The researchers noted that assaults which occurred in the street or in clubs or discotheques were unlikely to be recorded by the police. Overall, assaults on female victims were even less likely to be recorded than were assaults on males, again reflecting the down-playing of 'domestic' violence.

Just as a greater readiness to report assault probably accounts for some part of the rise in the official figures, it is likely that a greater police willingness to record assaults upon 'unpromising' victims has also contributed (Mayhew *et al.* 1993: 22). In Bristol, for example, each of the three police divisions which cover the city now records about a thousand complaints of 'domestic' assault each year (Cunningham 1990). This, in the words of a local Detective Chief Inspector, reflects a policy decision taken within the police force in 1988 'to intervene, rather than to ignore most complaints' (Cunningham 1990).

While there is good reason to suppose that certain categories of assault are more likely to be reported than hitherto and, having been reported, are more likely to be recorded by the police, we should not assume that the official record, even now, provides anything approaching a true picture. The disincentives to reporting and recording are too strong for that to be the case.[14] This encourages a search for alternative measures, notably the various *crime surveys* which have proved such a powerful tool in calculating the true level of criminal activity. On the basis of these data it has been estimated that only a quarter of criminal offences find their way on to police records. Furthermore, the rate of non-recording appears to be highest in relation to assaults and thefts from the person (Sparks *et al.* 1977: 157). The 1982 British Crime Survey suggested that only 23 per cent of violent offences and 11 per cent of robberies appeared in police crime records (Hough and Mayhew 1983). Latest British Crime Survey figures suggest that 17 per cent of robberies and 20 per cent of woundings are recorded by the police, compared with an 86 per cent recording rate for theft of motor vehicles.[15] This is consistent with survey data from other countries: the strongest correspondence between survey figures and offences recorded by the police is in relation to vehicle theft; there is a moderate correspondence for burglary; and a very poor correspondence for assault.[16]

As well as providing a truer measure of criminal activity, surveys offer an alternative means of comparing crime levels in different countries. One technique involves conducting victim surveys by telephone at the same time in several countries, with the same questions being asked. This has revealed England and Wales to have one of the lowest rates of non-sexual assault, well behind Australia and the USA.[17] Surveys also provide an alternative means of calculating *trends* in violent conduct, with the latest figures being compared with results for previous years. Overall, violent crime recorded by the British Crime Surveys rose by 8 per cent between the two surveys of 1982 and 1988,[18] while the 1992 survey revealed a further increase. The number of woundings rose from 507,000 in 1982 to 626,000 in 1992 – an increase of 12 per cent, while the number of common assaults rose from 1,402,000 to 1,757,000 – an increase of 25 per cent.[19]

It has been acknowledged, not least by the Home Office researchers principally responsible for the British Crime Surveys, that surveys have many limitations when it comes to calculating the level of violent crime (Hough 1991). Many assaults, Hough suggests, will not be defined by the victim as criminal because they take place in the domestic sphere. Non-domestic incidents may likewise not be defined as criminal even though an offence has clearly been committed. The problem with assault, as compared with an offence such as burglary, is that respondents will apply different criteria when answering so-called 'screen' questions such as: 'Has anyone hit or attacked you in any way?'. A related problem is to be found in the 'events' orientation of crime surveys. This assumes that infringements of the law are discrete incidents. But, Hough suggests, some violent offences are better conceptualised as processes rather than events. This is particularly true, it might be thought, of 'domestic' assault. And indeed it has been claimed that up to 25 per cent of women have been struck by their partner.[20] It has also been suggested that better educated respondents are more likely to report an assault because they have a lower tolerance of this type of offence and are more likely, therefore, to regard it as having crossed the 'crime' threshold (Mayhew *et al*. 1989: 5). If it is accepted that people differ in their attitudes towards violence, this creates problems for any attempt to measure the extent of violence by means of survey techniques. It has been suggested, for example, that middle-class men are more likely to be upset by violence than are their working-class counterparts, and that many 'assaults' are in fact minor fracas between young men which cause no great distress to the participants or to anyone else. These are matters which we shall explore in this book, but we can say immediately that it is wrong to suppose that there is widespread tolerance of violence on the part of assault victims, or that assaults not reported to the police generally involve incidents which might be characterised as 'six of one and half-a-dozen of the other'. In order to explore these questions properly we have to go beyond survey data. Even in terms of simple counting, it is necessary to study *behaviour* rather than to rely on self-reporting on the one hand or police-defined samples of victims on the other.

One measure of behaviour is the deliberate infliction of injury, and this has led researchers to attempt to measure the incidence of assault by reference to the Accident and Emergency (A & E) Department record of assault victims admitted to hospital for treatment. Shepherd *et al*. (1989) make the case for utilising this data source. They observe that the recording of violent offences by hospitals depends on the presence of injuries perceived to require treatment, rather than on victims' perception that a crime has been committed. Other advantages are that victims may be interviewed shortly after injury; that A & E Departments serve well-defined communities; and that hospitals are independent of the police. A disadvantage of this method of recording is that even the seriously injured may decide *not* to attend for treatment – may even be prevented or deterred from doing so by their assailant. But that is a problem common to the police record also. In fact the population of victims seeking hospital treatment may be largely distinct from that known to the police, and distinct also from that which is recorded in the various crime surveys. This is reflected in British Crime Survey data suggesting that most crimes of violence do not result in serious physical injury. The 1984 survey revealed that in only 12 per cent of assaults did the victim seek professional medical attention (Hough and Mayhew 1985), while the 1988 survey indicated that in respect of the more serious offence of wounding only 30 per cent of victims sought medical treatment (Mayhew *et al.* 1989: 37).

By virtue of their providing a partially distinct sample of assault victims, A & E Department records also provide an alternative measure of *trends* in violent conduct, and one that is not contaminated by changes in reporting behaviour or an increased police presence. Thus Shepherd *et al.* (1993) report, on the basis of hospital data gathered in Bristol, that the incidence of intentional injury for which treatment was sought at the local A & E Department reached a peak in 1983 and has not increased since. This finding is markedly at variance with the picture presented by police crime statistics. It may be that hospital data, while deficient in many respects, provide a better indicator of trends in violent conduct than do police records. A & E Departments may, at the very least, provide a better measure of *assaults occasioning significant injury* than do either police records or crime surveys; on the other hand, they are unlikely to provide an accurate measure of less serious violence.

A DIFFERENT KIND OF MONITORING

Gottfredson has suggested that 'because of the rarity and clustering of serious criminal victimisation. . .' crime surveys such as the ones now being conducted on a regular basis by the Home Office are not the best way to study the circumstances surrounding serious offences. He identifies 'a particular need to "flesh out" the situational aspects of criminal events' (Gottfredson 1984: 31). Sparks *et al.* were likewise alive to the limitations of victim studies such as their own and recommended further projects which would follow incidents through the justice system, starting at the earliest possible moment:

> In this way it would be possible to obtain a more complete picture of both the police and the public's reaction to crime incidents of various kinds, and to gain a better knowledge of the factors which lead some incidents to be settled informally without being recorded in police statistics of crime.
>
> (Sparks *et al.* 1977: 233).

That is indeed what we have attempted to do. A study of this kind enables the researcher to explore the possibility that even self-report studies arrive at an under-representation of the true level of crime. It also enables her to examine how victims (or apparent victims) understand their experience. It may be, for example, that some quite serious offences are not defined (by the victim) as criminal at all, but as 'six of one and half-a-dozen of the other', or as arising from a misunderstanding, or as being reasonable (and non-culpable) in all the circumstances. A major advantage of studying 'behaviour' rather than 'crime' is that we can then explore this question of the way in which victims define what has happened to them (for example, whether they had been engaged in a fight, or had suffered an assault). We are also able to see how victims reach a conclusion as to appropriate punishment, or remedy. This is impossible if one adopts the more usual approach of taking a group of offences which are being processed through the criminal courts. First, as we have seen, much 'crime' is unreported. Second, behaviour defined as criminal comprises only part of that which *could* be so defined. If we can understand what determines whether or not criminal behaviour becomes 'crime', we should have a better grasp of the real world than if we merely study the police, the Crown Prosecution Service, and the courts.

So it was that we decided to make a start outside the justice system. Our chosen starting point, for the purpose of the research underpinning this book, was the Accident and Emergency Department of a large city centre hospital. It is true of course that not all victims of violence report to an A & E Department. Indeed, it is likely that the majority do not. Nevertheless an A & E Department provides an excellent context in which to try to understand violence – especially, perhaps, violence leading to serious injury. It enabled us to secure a sample of assault victims which had not been filtered, nor the victims' status defined, by criminal justice agencies. The cases cannot be said to be representative of *all* 'assaults' (however assault is defined) and so from a survey perspective one might have reservations, but we cannot think of a better way of getting to grips with the issues surrounding criminalisation. Our study enabled us to gain a full picture of victims, of their 'story', and of any subsequent engagement between this story and the criminal justice process. This is far removed from the 'analysis of criminal statistics and the study of law reports' which one eminent judicial figure, now retired, has concluded to be the province of academic criminologists.[21]

RESEARCH METHOD

The task of identifying assault victims who attend for treatment at an Accident and Emergency Department is assisted by the fact that 'assault' is one of the causes of injury identified by reception staff. Nonetheless, problems remain. As we have said, 'assault' has various technical, legal definitions as well as a lay meaning. We were bound in the first instance to rely on the self-definition of patients. This was acceptable as far as we were concerned because the lay definition of assault tends to coincide with our own area of criminological interest – that is to say, it excludes 'corporate' violence or violence that is entirely accidental. The extent to which an assailant *intends* to inflict harm is a point at issue in many criminal trials,[22] and of course we would not have wished to exclude cases (perhaps the majority of assaults) in which there is room for argument concerning whether the assailant intended to inflict the degree of harm suffered by the victim, but we were not concerned with cases in which harm was entirely unforeseen. Nor would we have wished to include 'corporate' violence within our sampling net. This is despite the fact that, in 1991/2, 295 people were killed at work in violent incidents, while in the same year there were reports of 165,713 workers sustaining serious injuries at their workplace (Clarkson and Keating 1994: 234). The question of whether these 'accidents' should be responded to as crimes is considered at some length in criminal law texts, but since corporate violence, so-called, does not raise the same issues of processing as does interpersonal violence we were content that it be excluded from our study.

It should be clear from the above that we did not assume any close correspondence between a victim's account of his or her experience and the various legal definitions of assault. Indeed, for the purpose of our study these legal definitions were largely ignored. For example, we did not trouble ourselves, when drawing our case sample, with such questions as: 'was the assailant deemed to have been acting in self-defence?' It might be thought that once we allow ourselves to depart from some 'objective' standard such as that provided by the criminal law we risk drifting rudderlessly over an ocean without end. But we were content to take the victim's definition as our starting point because, as we have said, we wanted to explore perceptions and definitions of assault and then to study criminalisation against this background.

We approached patients either during their initial attendance at the A & E Department, or while they received in-patient treatment, or when they returned for subsequent out-patient treatment, or by letter. Following our initial contact, and usually within a few days or weeks of the assault, we spent approximately an hour with each victim, discussing as fully as possible the circumstances of the assault, their attitude towards criminalisation, and their reflections on what had happened to them and its implications in the longer term. Where the assault *had* been reported to the police we interviewed the officer principally concerned and, where prosecution followed, we observed all court proceedings. A fuller account of our research methodology is given in Appendix A.

One further point needs to be made about our research method. Research which takes the victim as its starting point is inevitably *victim-centred*. It is true of almost all social research that the researcher's perceptions, and indeed the research 'findings', will be significantly affected by decisions as to which set of actors to approach for information. The criminal justice system is concerned primarily with the processing of *offenders*. Much criminological research also has the offender as its focus. Our study is different: we started with the victim and we rarely spoke to the alleged assailant. This makes a difference to the way we view the criminalisation of assault. It means, for example, that we may be less sensitive to issues of suspect rights than if we had interviewed offenders, and less inclined also to challenge the injured person's version of events. It is as well for researchers always to recognise that they are not presented with the plain unvarnished truth; in situations of conflict, and perhaps especially where there is violence, a great deal depends on who is telling the tale. This is the basis of much of the criticism of crime surveys: Sparks *et al.*, when considering questions of victim precipitation of violence or proneness to victimisation, observe that victim surveys, which place heavy reliance upon victims' own accounts, can make but a limited contribution:

> in our opinion such retrospective and one-sided accounts of violent interaction must always be of limited value, at least unless very special interviewing techniques are used.
>
> (Sparks *et al.* 1977: 99–100)

We have done our best to surmount this problem by adopting a multi-layered approach which involved our interviewing police officers as well as victims, and then following this up with court observation, but we nonetheless concede that in many instances the information available to us was, at best, partial. This indeed bears on one of our key themes, outlined below.

Public and private purposes in prosecuting assault

Examining assaults in the way we did led us to view criminal prosecution in a new light, as presenting practical problems and theoretical inconsistencies which have received scant attention in the criminological literature. We might start from the fact that in some 57 per cent of assaults recorded by the 1992 British Crime Survey, victim and assailant were known to one another at least casually (Mayhew *et al.* 1993: 88). It follows that in order to understand violence one must view it in context, as perhaps one of a series of critical events involving people who have a personal relationship of some kind, a relationship often marked by an acute imbalance of power. This relationship tends to be 'private' in that it is in large part hidden from public view. If an assault is reported to the police and prosecuted through the courts there is a sense in which it is transferred to the public realm; but this transfer is problematic for three reasons: first, the prior personal relationship, if one exists, is likely to continue in some form thus making it extremely difficult for the assault victim to commit himself or herself to criminal proceedings; second, in the course of those criminal proceedings the assault is likely to be excised from its context, or if an attempt at contextualisation is made it is almost bound to be both inadequate and controversial; and third, the *purposes* reflected in the practice of lawyers and courts are in large part 'public' or symbolic purposes: criminal justice is not geared to redressing private wrongs.

This central theme – the difficulty of translating assault from the private to the public realm and the confusion of purpose evident in current attempts to achieve this – can be further developed under the following heads:

- the difficulty in penetrating character or events and, therefore, in discharging the probative burden
- the significance of prior personal relationships
- the relationship between seriousness and criminalisation
- the clash between private and public purposes.

The difficulty in penetrating character or events and, therefore, in discharging the probative burden

Each assault is a story, but a story which could be told in many different ways. This is a problem for the researcher, and a problem also for the court. Any outsider, whether independent observer or trier of fact, will experience difficulty in penetrating a violent incident, especially given the character and lifestyle of some of those involved. In some of the cases which we followed our sense of the anatomy of the event was quite firm; but in others there was considerable room for doubt. This might arise from confusions in the victim's own account (possibly as a result of his or her having been drunk at the time), or from discrepancies between the victim's story and the accounts offered by witnesses.

A number of factors may contribute to the outsider's instinct that he or she has failed fully to understand the event. In some of the cases which we followed the victim was clearly confused, possibly as a result of habitual alcoholism and/or mental impairment. Where such a person had been assaulted on a more or less regular basis it was virtually impossible to unravel one particular incident. In other cases it seemed probable that victims wished to conceal certain matters (such as their own propensity for violent conduct, or the extent to which they had provoked their assailant) or to misrepresent themselves (for example, as having been more co-operative with the police than was in fact the case). Other interviews had a shadowy quality because it was difficult to penetrate the lifestyle of our informant, or to understand the nature of the relationship between 'victim' and 'assailant'. The world of some victims was so foreign to the interviewer that it was difficult to interpret their talk, or to get any real sense of their mental landscape. In other instances the actors in the drama presented starkly conflicting accounts: our interviews with police officers and, even more so, our attendance at court commonly alerted us to such discrepancies. There were also a few cases where the *police* construction of events was at odds with the victim's own account: for example, in one case we could not be sure whether the 'victim' had been assaulted or whether, as the police alleged, he had staged the attack (by hitting himself over the head with a breeze block) in order to conceal a robbery.

The researcher's problems are of a different order to those faced by the police, CPS, or court, but there is a sense in which everyone is struggling with the same problem, namely to achieve a reliable reconstruction of what may have been a complex event. The task of the prosecuting authorities is to establish the guilt of the defendant, not to bring out all the nuances of that event. Accordingly, the prosecution process is likely to idealise the victim as innocent, passive, and not contributing in any material way to his or her own victimisation (Shapland *et al.* 1985: 66). As Shapland and her colleagues observe, this image of the innocent victim tends to be sharply challenged at the criminal trial. The job of defence counsel is to supply a rival explanation of the events which gave rise to the charge (Rock 1993: 33). The defence case does not need to be as 'solid' as that of the prosecution. Merely by under-mining the impression conveyed by prosecution witnesses, counsel for the defence may persuade the jury that they cannot 'without a shadow of a doubt' accept the prosecution account. It might emerge, for example, that the victim's recollection of events leading up to the assault was somewhat hazy. By highlighting apparent inconsistencies in witness accounts concerning peripheral matters the defence might cast doubt upon the victim's ability to recall the assault itself. The adversarial nature of the proceedings could transform what on paper (and from the victim's earlier account to us) appeared cut and dried into something far less certain. Trials in which (from our privileged position) there appeared no doubt that the defendant had caused some injury to the victim might nonetheless raise doubts about the prosecution case in the mind of the observer. If this can be so in cases which, beforehand, appear 'open and shut', how much more vulnerable are those prosecutions in which the complainant or other witnesses are of dubious status?

The relationship between seriousness and criminalisation

One may conceive the criminalisation of assault as a process of attrition, with a significant 'drop-out' rate at each successive stage. This can be illustrated by reference to the ninety-three assault victims whom we identified after they had sought treatment at a hospital Accident and Emergency Department. Figure 1.1 reveals the 'progress' of these ninety-three cases. Ninety-three assaults produced twenty-two convictions. The main 'drop-out' points were: (a) through the police not being informed of an incident in the first instance (nineteen cases); (b) through there being no formal 'complaint' in some of those cases in which the assault was brought to police attention (twenty cases); and (c) through the police being unable to identify the assailant or amass sufficient evidence against him (sixteen cases). There was also a significant failure rate later in the process, at the point when cases were brought to court, principally through victims' failure to sustain a commitment to the prosecution effort.

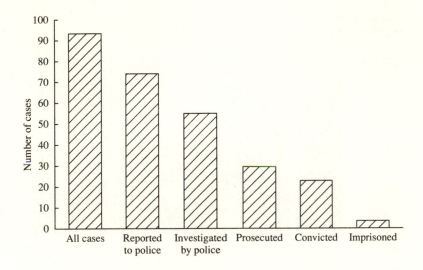

Figure 1.1 The extent of criminalisation among our sample of assault cases

This attrition rate is perhaps unremarkable in itself. But what is certainly noteworthy, and demanding of explanation, is that there appears to be almost a random relationship between *seriousness*, as we defined it, and the reporting, investigation, and prosecution of assault. At the very least there is no simple linear relationship between seriousness on the one hand and criminalisation on the other. This is apparent from Figure 1.2, in which is shown the extent of criminalisation among the ninety-three assaults which we followed, placed in our own rank order of 'seriousness', the most serious cases being on the left, the most trivial on the right.[23]

It is true that most (although not all) very grave assaults are reported, investigated, and (assuming detection) prosecuted, but apart from the very top end of the scale the relationship between seriousness and criminalisation is remarkable for the fact that there is *no* relationship, at least as far as we were able to determine. Nor is failure to convict in serious cases always accounted for by a failure to identify the assailant, or by lack of evidence. With the exception of violence arising in pubs, clubs, or on the street, detection is not in itself the main problem. The police may be called to an assault to find 'victim' and 'assailant' still at the scene. In many cases the two parties are known to one another. But while this makes detection apparently straightforward, it may not assist prosecution.

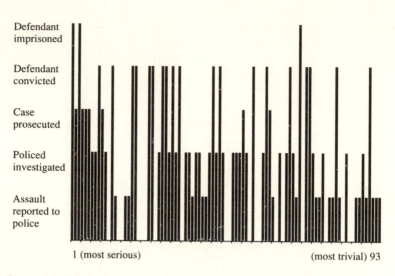

Figure 1.2 Criminalisation of assault cases matched against seriousness of injury

The importance of prior personal relationships

It is one of our tasks in this book to try to explain the apparently almost random relationship which we observe between culpability and harm on the one hand and conviction and punishment on the other. Of particular significance in this context is the burden of the prosecution process upon assault victims at every stage, including initial reporting, and the extreme vulnerability of those victims who have a continuing relationship with their assailant. Assaults by strangers are difficult to detect; assaults by acquaintances, or intimates, present few problems of detection but can nonetheless be extremely difficult to prosecute. This reflects one of our central themes – that each assault needs to be viewed in context. A key element in that context, affecting both the victim's definition of the assailant's behaviour and his or her inclination to report the matter to the police, is the fact of a prior personal relationship. Much of the data concerning prior relationships have been in relation to homicides, a high proportion of which involve friends, relatives, or acquaintances. Prior relationships feature in a lower proportion of non-homicidal assaults, but this may be because assaults by family members or friends are less likely than other assaults to be brought to the attention of the prosecuting authorities. The 1984 British Crime Survey indicated that some 18 per cent of assaults were 'domestic' – that is, perpetrated by a partner, ex-partner, or other household member, while in approximately 50 per cent of cases (in total) victim and offender were known to each other (Hough and Mayhew 1985: 9). The survey conducted by Sparks *et al.* (1977) produced similar findings: 47 per cent of assaults were committed by family members or acquaintances. Thirty-seven of the ninety-three assault victims whose cases we followed knew their assailant well. Seventeen (18 per cent) had been assaulted by partners or by fellow family members. Fifteen out of twenty-two women (68 per cent) had been assaulted by their sexual partner or by another member of their family. Male victims, on the other hand, were assaulted by their partners or by other family members in just two out of seventy-one cases (3 per cent).

Where the victim is involved in a family or sexual relationship with the assailant, or simply inhabiting the same social milieu, the decision to initiate criminal proceedings may carry with it all the baggage of a disrupted relationship, loss of face, risk of exposing the private realm to the public gaze, and the prospect of emotional blackmail and, perhaps, further physical harm. As far as our own study was concerned, it seemed that this was true of most cases in which there was a reasonable prospect of detection. *Fear of reprisals*, especially, is a major factor in non-reporting. Whenever victim and assailant have an on-going relationship, whether as partners, family members, or *habitués* of a common social environment, it may be felt that neither the police nor the courts will be able to prevent further attacks or other threatening behaviour. The key to understanding the difficulties inherent in prosecuting assault is to understand the relationship between victim and assailant. The failure to prosecute effectively is not principally attributable to problems of detection, but rather to the fact that many victims remain trapped in their assailant's web of power.

The clash between private and public purposes

It is essential, in seeking to understand the criminalisation of assault, to ask whose purposes are being served at each stage in the process. In noting that many assault victims find it difficult to cooperate with the prosecuting authorities we are making implicit acknowledgement of the fact that criminal prosecution may do little to assist the victim – may even do him or her harm – while the victim's own needs, say for protection from further violence, may not be met. The police might say that they act on behalf of the victim, but there is a sense in which they use the victim in furtherance of their main objective, which is to secure the conviction of the offender. It is true that the assailant will seldom be prosecuted unless the victim is shown to be committed to the process, but is that necessarily the reason he or she went to the police in the first instance? Does prosecution offer anything to the victim beyond the prospect of further pain – this time at the hands of 'authority'?[24]

There was a time when the above question might have been answered quite straightforwardly in the negative. Many commentators have remarked upon the justice system's preoccupation with the offender (see, for example, McDonald 1976: 18–27), while others have noted the practical difficulties created for the prosecution by the idealisation of the victim as innocent, passive, and having no significant prior relationship with the defendant (Shapland *et al.* 1985). There has subsequently been a reaction against criminological analyses which focused exclusively upon the offender, and a shift in criminological interest away from the crime control/due process debates of the 1960s in which the victim was largely ignored (Miers 1992). McDonald has analysed the sudden inter-est in 'victimology' in terms of the 'convergence of the interests of scholars, activists, and public officials who are concerned with the plight of different kinds of victim' – for example, the elderly, children, and victims of sexual offences (McDonald 1976: 18–27). Had the author been writing a few years later he would no doubt have referred also to victims of 'domestic' violence. As Miers has observed, expressed con-cern for the interests of crime victims 'constitutes an almost unassailable moral position' (Miers 1992), but this apparent unanimity conceals starkly contrasting analyses and agendas for reform (Miers 1992). Proponents of 'victims' rights' straddle the political spectrum, with this being a convenient rallying cry for those whose primary purpose is to achieve more severe punishment for offenders. There is no single reform programme which would command widespread support.

Victimology, if this is defined as the study of those on the receiving end of crime, can appear rather uninteresting. This is because crime victims do not form any kind of coherent group. Some people are victimised on a more or less regular basis, and in very disabling ways; for others this is an occasional, apparently chance experience. Some victims are themselves offenders, and so on. One indication of the inherently unsatisfactory nature of victimology as a discipline is the fact that even those studies which claim to be about victims are quite fre-quently more concerned with victims' attitude towards offenders than they are with the victim's own experience. This certainly suggests that we find victims a good deal less interesting than we do offenders. And it is true that, taken *en masse*, victims can appear of greater interest to the moral entrepreneur than they are to the sociologist or the policy-maker. What is there to do once we have expressed our compassion and indignation?

But victims are not uninteresting if their victimisation is placed in the context of their life as a whole, which often means locating it within a key relationship. If assault is part of a pattern in people's lives, then it is important to explore the relationships out of which the violence springs. In this way, also, one can begin to understand from the victim's perspective the significance of the various stages of criminalisation. What is the point of going to the police? What are the likely consequences of giving evidence against their assailant? And so on. Having done that one may be in a position to review the dominant models of criminal justice within which the victim's interest is meant to be subsumed. We will describe how victims' perception of the harm suffered is frequently not matched by legal definitions, while conduct of the case by the police and the presentation of these matters in court often fails to reflect the victim's own account. As a result, the relationship between the victim's needs and intentions in reporting an act of violence and the criminal justice outcome is a complex one in which the legal process frequently and for a variety of reasons inflicts further harm on the person whom it might be thought designed to protect (Miers 1992).

If we accept, as most academic commentators and practitioners do accept, that the main purpose of criminal proceedings is to enable the state to respond to a wrong done to itself, then neglect of the victim's interest may be seen as regrettable, but understandable and perhaps inevitable. If however we recognise the system's absolute reliance upon victims – not only as reporters, but as staunch complainants and witnesses – we may begin to perceive a remarkable disjunction between this absolute reliance upon victims as the 'trigger' of criminalisation and the subsequent rigorous adherence to an offence against society model. To what extent can this model be sustained given the premium placed upon victim co-operation and commitment to the process? *Ought* it to be sustained? And to what extent is it possible for the justice system to address private harm even as it engages in symbolic denunciation of wrongdoing?

Chapter 2

The reality of assault

In this chapter we shall consider who is most at risk of assault; second, we shall describe the range of circumstances in which people are assaulted; and third we shall try to convey something of the reality of that experience. An obvious starting point is with a simple numerical analysis of known assault victims by sex, age and race.

SEX

As far as the sex of victims is concerned, police records and survey data suggest that men are at least twice as likely to be assaulted as are women (Sparks *et al*. 1977; Davidoff and Dowds 1989). There is an even higher proportion of male victims in respect of assaults causing more serious injury (1988 British Crime Survey; Davidoff and Greenhorn 1991). On the other hand, a greater number of women report that they have been assaulted on more than one occasion (Sparks *et al*. 1977: 83). One must also make a sharp distinction between the 'public' and 'private' spheres. Assaults are overwhelmingly perpetrated by men. Men in public use violence against other males, whom they may not know. In private they assault women, whom they *do* know.

British Crime Survey data, supported by other research studies in this country and in the USA, suggest that the paradigm victim of personal violence is the young male, although it is necessary to bear in mind the probable high rate of under-reporting of violence in the home and the consequent under-recording of female victimisation. The Home Office researchers responsible for the various British Crime Surveys have acknowledged that their method of surveying victims is unlikely to reveal the true extent of crimes against women (Mayhew *et al*. 1993: 5). One message of victimisation surveys is that the closer the relationship between offender and victim, the less likely it is that the offence will be reported (Moonman 1987; Strauss *et al*. 1980). One must enter the same reservations in respect of hospital data. For example, Shepherd's survey of Accident and Emergency Department records found that only 16 per cent of assault victims were female (Shepherd 1990a). In fact this is a lower percentage of female victims than among our own hospital-based sample: we noted that of 376 assault victims referred to the Bristol Royal Infirmary A & E Department in March and April 1990, 102 were female (27 per cent), while the hospital-derived sample of ninety-three victims whose cases we followed through the justice system included twenty-two women (24 per cent). Again we might surmise that the victim of 'private' violence is less likely to seek treatment; or, if the victim does go to hospital, he or she may not give a true account of the cause of injuries. In short, all attempts at quantifying assault are bedevilled by the likely under-reporting of violence by men against women in the home. This in turn reflects the fact that 'domestic' violence tends to be viewed as a social and psychological problem rather than, primarily, as a criminal matter. It has been suggested that those who work in this area (police, lawyers, magistrates, court staff and judiciary) may 'deter applicants from pursuing their proceedings . . . if their reactions are affected by particular perceptions of male and female roles or an ambivalence about the propriety of legal or police intervention within the family' (Law Commission 1992).

Use of the term 'domestic' is revealing in itself. Employed in connection with assault, it conjures up a variety of images and associations – and therein lies its true significance. Police and prosecutor use of this term is not intended to imply any precise definition of the relationship between victim and assailant beyond the implication that it has (or had) some element of intimacy. The assault in question need not be upon a sexual partner for it to be referred to by the investigating police officer as 'having something of the domestic about it', or 'semi-domestic', or 'a bit domesticky'. It seemed to us that as well as implying that the parties had some kind of prior personal relationship – if only as friends, acquaintances, or fellow family members – police officers used the term 'domestic' as a coded reference to the response which the incident elicited from them and from their sense that the parties' relationship was *predictive of the case's anticipated career*, notably in the expectation that the victim would prove an unreliable complainant.

AGE

The age profile of assault victims can be stated with greater confidence than can breakdown by sex, although here again allowance must be made for the largely hidden phenomenon of domestic assault and the different age profile which might result were more of these cases to be included. Survey data suggest that 16–29 year olds are most at risk, with 68 per cent of all assaults being committed against persons in this age group (Mayhew *et al.* 1993: 127). Surveys in the USA reveal a victimisation peak among those in the 16–19 age group, with a progressive decline with increasing age (Hindelang *et al.* 1978). The elderly have by far the lowest risk of assault (Mawby 1988). This finding was deemed newsworthy when the first British Crime Survey was published, principally because of the extent to which the British press had misidentified the elderly as primary targets of violent crime. Even when their reduced exposure to risk is taken into account, victimisation rates for the elderly appear to be low. It is noteworthy, however, that assault victims aged over 50 appear much less inclined to report the incident to the police (Sparks *et al.* 1977), reminding us once again that police records of assault and, to a lesser extent, survey data can each seriously mislead. Hospital records indicate a somewhat older age profile for assault victims, with Shepherd's study (1990a) suggesting a mean age of 26/27, while our own survey of 376 assault victims found that 50 per cent were in their twenties and 15 per cent were aged over 40. We also found that the older age groups included a higher proportion of female victims: women comprised 22 per cent of the under-20 age category; 25 per cent of those aged 20–30; and 34 per cent of victims aged over 30.

RACE

The third readily quantifiable measure is that of race. On the whole, blacks are significantly more likely to be assaulted than are whites (Sparks *et al.* 1977). The 1988 British Crime Survey indicated that 3 per cent of whites were assaulted over the recall period, compared with 7 per cent of African–Caribbeans and 4 per cent of Asians.[1] It would appear also that African–Caribbeans and Asians were more likely to have been assaulted on more than one occasion. (Our hospital-derived sample of ninety-two assault victims is unrepresentative in this respect since it comprised eighty-eight whites, two African-Caribbeans and two Asians.[2]) If we accept that African–Caribbeans and, to a lesser extent, Asians are more likely to be assaulted than are whites, this is probably related to other environmental disadvantages suffered by these groups, including inner city residence, poor housing, and leisure time spent in potentially dangerous locations. Also, African–Caribbeans in this country are typically younger than whites and more likely to have a single lifestyle.

It would appear that a high proportion of assaults are *intra-racial*. Sparks *et al*. (1977) found that 71.6 per cent of white victims had white assailants, while 68.8 per cent of black victims had black assailants. This is not borne out by our own study which comprised few non-white victims but a high proportion of non-white assailants. In fact, in relation to these ninety-three incidents, sixty-one assailants were said to be white (66 per cent); twenty-four were said to be African–Caribbean (26 per cent); one was Asian; and in eight cases the assailant's race was un-known. We are loath to attach much significance to this finding given the obvious risk that non-white victims were under-represented in our hospital-based sample. It is also important to recognise that there is not always a clear-cut distinction between 'victim' and 'offender': had we talked to some alleged assailants we might have been prepared to re-classify them as victims. In any event the high proportion of black assailants should not come as a surprise: the conditions that, according to most studies, generate a high proportion of black victims are likely also to generate black assailants – that is to say, the various environmental disadvantages listed above, plus the fact of a relatively youthful population which is inclined to spend its leisure time in dangerous locations (Shepherd 1990a).

LIFESTYLE

Early research on victimisation concentrated on fixed characteristics such as age, sex and socio-economic group. This has tended to be replaced by 'lifestyle' models of victimisation which focus on *behaviour* – how often a person goes out at night, to what locations, with which companions, leading to the consumption of how much alcohol, and so on (Levi 1994: 301). A young man in search of drink and entertainment in a city centre pub or club on a Friday or Saturday night is exposed to a risk of violence which the rest of us, by virtue of our age, sobriety, decorum and unexciting social pursuits, have no reason to contemplate. Accordingly, a lifestyle or 'exposure' model is now broadly accepted as a measure of susceptibility to victimisation. Sparks *et al*. (1977: 105) observed that victims of violence were likely to be persons 'who lead reasonably active social lives. Further, they are much more likely to be attacked by a friend, acquaintance, or family member than by a stranger; and in many cases they will have provoked or induced the crime by their own actions'. Gottfredson (1981), in a study not confined to violent offences, concluded that the risks of victimisation were higher for young, male, single people. This was especially true of those who live in the inner cities, go out at night, use public transport, consume alcohol on a regular basis, are themselves offenders, and who suffer a variety of other, non-criminal victimisations. These predictors suggest that there are, broadly, two kinds of victim of public violence: the person who chooses a particular form of leisure activity, namely, drinking in a crowded public place; and the person whose lifestyle is such that he or she has little chance of avoiding violence. The person who lives in poor housing or on the street, who is alcoholic, who lives among alcoholics or people suffering from mental disorder, is liable to all manner of victimisation including, specifically, assault (Zedner 1994: 1214). Such a person bears a disproportionate part of the burden of threatened or actual physical violence which, for many of us, may be considered virtually negligible (see, for a comparable in-depth study of repeated victimisation, Genn 1988). As Miers observes, 'on the margins of English urban society there are people who suffer almost continuous criminal victimisation . . . and the mere recording of criminal events . . . tells us little about the quality, or rather lack of quality, of their lives' (Miers 1992).

One such habitual victim whom we observed in the course of our own study, Royston Kilmore (44)[3] was a homeless, unemployed alcoholic who sought accommodation and food at the Bristol city centre night shelter. The violence which he had suffered in this one instance was, by his account, part of a pattern of behaviour characterised by heavy drinking, baiting by his companions, and physical confrontation. It was the action of the night shelter staff which brought this incident to the attention of the police. But many other assaults, taking place in the open, on the street, or in underpasses, go unrecorded. Such behaviour cannot readily be dealt with by the court and it washes around the feet of the police without actually trickling into their shoes (or their files). This man was one of several 'down and outs' who figured in our research sample as victims but whom we suspected were capable of inflicting violence as well as suffering it. Indeed, their categorisation as either 'victim' or 'offender' may be arbitrary and virtually meaningless. Men who have been driven to adopt this lifestyle, and who are habitually drunk, tend to be of volatile disposition. One described himself as 'very panicky and neurotic'. We had no doubt that he could both provoke violence and inflict it.

Other habitual victims appeared relatively peaceable, but their vulnerability lay in their oppressed circumstances. Dave Knowles (41), a street newspaper seller, told us that the police kept an eye on him because he was 'very vulnerable to attacks'. Given his mental confusion, his heavy drinking, and his job which entailed carrying money about hostile streets, he was forever at risk. Tom Robinson (14), a south Somerset man, was charged with assaulting his wife and bailed to cool his heels in a St Paul's hostel over the New Year. A confirmed alcoholic, and drunk before he even set foot in Bristol, he fell victim to a violent neighbourhood on New Year's Eve. These men were typical of a significant minority of assault victims who owed their vulnerability to their marginal status. This marginality was frequently a product of alcoholism or mental impairment, but many other factors might contribute to their outsider status. We came to refer to some victims as 'outlaws' – a characterisation which reflected their adoption of a criminal or anti-social lifestyle which, at least in their own eyes, placed them beyond the protection of the criminal law. To take another example, Walter Bristow (16) was a heavy drug user with, by his own account, a formidable criminal record. Wanted by the police at the time of his assault, afraid of reprisals and living by force of circumstances in the St Paul's district of Bristol, he had no reason to report his assault of which there were in any event no witnesses. Although severely injured, he was more oppressed by the broad circumstances of his life (imprisonment; drug dependency; exposure to continued threat within the criminal underworld) than he was upset by this particular incident. His espousal of a criminal lifestyle appeared to have made him insensible to moral affront. In all, fifty-one out of the ninety-two victims whose cases we monitored (55 per cent) told us that they had been assaulted previously as an adult. Those who had suffered repeated assaults because of the oppressed circumstances in which they lived appeared older than the average: whereas crime survey data suggest that most assault victims fall within the 16–24 age band, our 'outlaws' were in their early thirties to late fifties.

PREDICTORS

Certain aspects of repeated victimisation are implicit in the above analysis and it is worth treating each with some care since they each contribute to the aetiology of assault. They are: the consumption of alcohol, whether by victim or offender; second, location; third, the victim's own criminality; and, finally, the victim's own role in precipitating the assault. We consider each of these in turn.

Alcohol and victimisation

Australian researchers have conducted a study of public drinking places in which violence is a recurring phenomenon and have concluded that there are 'violent drinking situations' (Tomsen *et al.* 1991). The key determinants of violence, the authors argue, are: (a) the type of customer; (b) the 'atmosphere' in the pub or club; (c) the amount of alcohol consumed; and (d) the behaviour of doormen. A preponderance of males led to sexual competitiveness so that, especially if the men were in identifiable groups and the groups were strangers to one another, violence was likely to follow. 'Atmosphere' was reflected in such matters as discomfort, excessive noise, and lack of space. Discomfort in turn led to faster drinking. Loud music was a factor in provoking violence but live *bands* (which offer entertainment) militated against. So the researchers identified boredom as another key factor underlying violent outbursts. Predictably, the more violent occasions were also marked by higher levels of drunkenness. Finally, edgy and aggressive bouncers (rather than bar staff) created a violence-prone atmosphere. Some doormen were obsessed with their own machismo and acted as if their employment gave them a licence to assault customers. In summary, according to these researchers, if you want to observe violence in public places you should go where you will find groups of male strangers, in circumstances of some physical discomfort, lacking entertainment, getting very drunk, and policed by aggressive and unreasonable bouncers.

This is consistent with the findings of our own research. There are certain readily identifiable pubs in the centre of Bristol in which large numbers of young people congregate together and drink too much. Nick Castle (56), a young man who worked as a barman in one of these places and who had had his nose broken by a customer, told us that he regarded them as a kind of proving ground. Customers were always 'on edge', either looking for trouble or waiting for it to happen. He believed that the violence was 'a lot to do with the age group', and also reflected the amount of drink ingested and the tension generated by having a great many bodies crammed together. It was the object of these establishments to try to cram as many people as possible into the available space. Bar staff were under constant pressure to serve drinks as quickly as possible. Because they were rushed off their feet they tended to be surly. Pubs and clubs such as this were dark, hot, and smoky. It was an atmosphere in which one positively anticipated fights breaking out.

Another element in pub and club violence is the bouncer culture within which some very aggressive young men find an outlet for their violent natures. Two of the most serious assaults which we studied were perpetrated by bouncers – and not just by the odd maverick, but by four to six men from two neighbouring establishments coming together to administer a sustained beating to one or more of their customers. In the Kevin Pilcher case (27) there was a minor precipitating cause – a few hostile words exchanged with another customer – followed by a group assault. This was also the pattern in the far more serious incident when Patrick Dashwood (3) and three friends who were in Bristol by reason of their work were set upon by up to six to eight 'bouncers' from two neighbouring establishments and subjected to a vicious attack which in one instance was life-threatening. Each of these affairs had a certain primitive clannish element to it, with the group responding, however implausibly, to an affront to one of their number.

It was instructive to discover this rather primitive Wild West scene operating in the heart of Bristol – as it does, we must assume, in other major cities. It is also noteworthy that while these locations appear to be breeding grounds for violence, the police, according to the assault victims whom we interviewed, are not much in evidence. It is an inhospitable environment for the police, and doubtless their presence would be welcomed neither by landlords nor by most customers, but the seriousness of some of the assaults which we monitored led us to question the appropriateness of permitting these establishments to be policed only by doormen who develop a mentality which can lead them to impose their own brand of summary justice upon customers. A spate of these incidents produced some police reaction – and associated press comment – in Bristol in 1992. A senior officer told magistrates attending the annual licensing session that the police were worried by the number of serious assaults involving door staff. They were not satisfied with the vetting procedures adopted by those agencies which provide bouncers; accordingly, the police were contemplating introducing their own training and monitoring scheme for doormen.

A third factor in generating a hostile environment may be the reluctance of some pub landlords to involve the police in bringing assailants to book – possibly because they wish to protect the reputation of their premises and also, perhaps, because they fear that they might lose their licence. (It is not only pub landlords who think like this: one assault victim whose case we followed worked at a Students' Union – he gave us to understand that his employers adopted the same policy.) The landlord of the premises which had seen a particularly brutal assault on Gary Atkinson (18) told the victim: 'As far as I'm concerned the matter is now finished with . . . we don't want no steward's inquiry down here'.

We asked Atkinson whether this indicated that the landlord was a somewhat unsavoury character, to which he replied: "A typical landlord . . . there's not a savoury landlord". Atkinson was not the only pub 'regular' to imply that his landlord preferred to control his premises with the aid of a few 'heavy' customers rather than resort to the police. Some of these arrangements might be informal, with the 'heavy' enjoying a status half-way between that of customer and doorman.

The fact that violence in pubs and clubs accounts for a significant proportion of all reported violent crime[4] suggests also that there is a link between alcohol in itself and the commission of violent offences[5] – and a link also between alcohol consumption and being on *the receiving end* of violence. Gottfredson, in an elaboration of the findings of the 1982 British Crime Survey, calculated that alcohol consumption was associated with an increased risk of victimisation across the range of criminal offences, with heavy drinkers being at greater risk than moderate drinkers, who in turn were at greater risk than occasional drinkers or abstainers (Gottfredson 1984). One American study found that nearly two-thirds of a prison population of assaulters had been drinking at the time of their offence, while another group of researchers, studying links between alcohol consumption and homicide, found that two-thirds of their sample of assailants *and 50 per cent of their victims* had been drinking immediately prior to the offence (Hodge 1993).

Hospital data likewise suggest a striking correlation between the consumption of alcohol and violent conduct. Australian researchers studying assault victims referred to a hospital casualty department noted, virtually as an aside, that in many instances both attacker and victim were drunk (Cuthbert *et al.* 1991). Similarly, Shepherd and colleagues at the Bristol Royal Infirmary compared a group of assault victims attending their A & E Department with a control group of friends or acquaintances who also attended the hospital but who had not suffered violence. They found that those who had been injured had consumed significantly more alcohol than their friends in the six hours leading up to the incident (Shepherd *et al.* 1990a). There is no doubt therefore that the consumption of alcohol in public places predisposes to violence. This applies particularly to young males who spend several evenings each week in noisy crowded places frequented almost exclusively by their own age group.

Our own study of 93 assaults confirmed the significance of alcohol as a trigger of assault. Indeed, we came to regard cases in which drink was *not* a factor as rather remarkable. Of our sample, 20 per cent had suffered violence in pubs or clubs: all of these victims had drunk a certain amount and many had been drinking heavily. In all, 33 per cent of our sample of victims admitted to having been severely affected by alcohol and/or drugs at the time of their assault; a further 26 per cent said they had been moderately affected; and 37 per cent told us that they had not been drinking or claimed that they had not drunk enough to affect their behaviour. It was more difficult for us to assess whether *the assailant* was drink-affected, but of those victims who claimed to be able to assess their assailant's degree of sobriety or intoxication ($n = 55$), 49 per cent thought that their assailant had been severely intoxicated and a further 13 per cent believed that that person had been moderately affected by alcohol. Thirty-nine victims claimed to know something of their assailant's pattern of alcohol consumption: of these, eight (21 per cent) considered their assailant to be alcohol-dependent and a further fourteen (36 per cent) reported that their assailant engaged in frequent, heavy, public drinking.

It seems that one effect of alcohol is to lead the drinker to interpret the words and actions of others as threatening, thereby increasing 'defensive activity' (Gustafson and Kallinen 1989). In other words, a drunken man may act aggressively when he believes himself to be behaving defensively. This is consistent with our own observations – as is illustrated by Bill Winter (93), a young man who first figured in our sample as a victim, or alleged victim, he having reported to hospital for treatment to a head wound. Having recently lost his girlfriend and his job, he had by his own account consumed £75 worth of alcohol in the course of the day. While waiting to be treated in the A & E Department of the Bristol Royal Infirmary Winter overheard (or mis-heard) a conversation between a couple whom he understood to be a remorseful husband and his battered wife. This triggered in our hero the desire, as he himself described it, 'to have a chat', so when the husband went to the toilet:

> I followed him into the toilet to have a chat with him and I went about it the wrong way and he started mouthing and went to hit me and I nutted him.

In this case we had no doubt that the husband was innocent of any aggressive action. But other assault victims probably contributed to their own victimisation in the sense that their judgement and self-protective instincts were impaired by drink. For example, Alex Thomas (75) made an attempt to deter a youth from destroying a notice-board outside a dental surgery. He said something to the effect of 'You're not going to get away with that!' whereupon he was punched several times. He conceded that he had been emboldened by drink:

I do feel that if I hadn't had a few drinks, I'd have been a little more cautious. Alternatively I might have been a little bit quicker on my feet in dodging the punch or seeing it coming, and in that sense I think you could say I did contribute, unfortunately.

Finally, we noted that violence between sexual partners or family members was frequently triggered by drinking on the part of one or both. In some cases it appeared that drinking was the root cause of the dispute: a son might turn upon the mother whose alcoholism offended him; a woman, herself drunk, might physically attack a partner whose heavy drinking threatened to break up their relationship. One young woman, Jane Bond (68), recalled the build-up to violence as follows:

That night I'd been drinking and drinking and drinking because it was my birthday, and I was drunk as a skunk.

According to her, her *partner's* drinking habits had already put pressure on their relationship. Previous violence had always been precipitated by his drinking. So drink was a factor not only in this particular incident, but in the build-up of resentment which lay behind it:

I hated him. All the hate came out, everything.

It would be simplistic to assert that such explosions of violence are 'caused' by drink. While it appears to be the case that alcohol consumed by both parties is a factor in many domestic assaults – as it is in many homicides (McHugh and Thompson 1991) – it may be that situational and interpersonal factors play at least an equal part. In other words, it may not simply be a matter of the man becoming violent when drunk, although we accept that this is a fair description of many 'domestic' assaults. As has been observed in relation to homicide:

Two individuals may be equally handicapped . . . the effect may be one of synergy rather than a simply additive effect. The social interactions in such situations may best be conceptualised as containing the potential for a downward spiral of misunderstandings.

(McHugh and Thompson 1991)

This is consistent with our own observations. Violence might follow a pattern of behaviour which had established itself through the couple's relationship, a pattern characterised by heavy drinking on both sides. Alice Smythe (61) told us that she drank to keep up with her partner:

Because if you're with someone who's drunk and you're not, you might as well be alone.

The violence only occurred, she said, when her partner had been drinking. This he did 'almost constantly', consuming thirty to forty pints of beer a week. She had suffered most from his violence when she herself drank:

A lot of the things that have happened have happened when I've gone too far, been too drunk to really have my wits about me.

This couple remained together, Smythe expressing a need for her partner despite the harm he had done her. She was trying to adopt a new technique ('switching off') for dealing with his drinking, but there was a continuing fear that the violence might recur:

I'm living from day to day . . . I dread it all starting again.

Another victim of 'domestic' violence, Helen Evans (22), told us that she became violent when drunk and that this in turn precipitated violence by her partner. Drink gave rise to the expression of deep hurts and grievances: the violence was then followed by calmer communication and expressed commitment to one another. She believed that if she could overcome her alcoholism she would no longer be at risk at the hands of her partner. From a feminist perspective this readiness to assume responsibility for one's own victimisation might be regarded as no more than a symptom of the subordination of women, and certainly in terms of real physical threat 'the problem' is one of *male* violence. We would nonetheless observe that alcohol often acts as a trigger to violence which has its roots in feelings of hurt and grievance lying at the heart of an intimate relationship – and that both parties may have these feelings, and both may drink.

Geography and victimisation[6]

Most British and North American research indicates that people who live in inner cities and other severely deprived urban areas are particularly vulnerable to most forms of personal victimisation, including assault (Gottfredson 1984: 8; Sparks *et al*. 1977). Those who spend a lot of time on the street, perhaps because of inadequate housing or unemployment, are at similarly high risk. Our own research bears this out. Certainly one can think of few better examples of being 'in the wrong place at the wrong time' than to find oneself in Bristol city centre on a Friday or Saturday night as closing time approaches, alcohol consumption rises, and the noise and overcrowding reach unbearable proportions. Many pubs in Bristol have occasional incidents of violence, but some experience them all the time. In King Street in the centre of Bristol respectable middle-class culture seekers come and go nightly, rubbing shoulders with those who find their entertainment in the fetid atmosphere of *The Black Dog*, while on St Augustine's Parade a tide of sensitive opera goers washes up against the flotsam and jetsam of *The Avenue* and similar establishments. To attend one of these places (the pubs, not the opera) is positively to anticipate violence breaking out.

Far more oppressive, one may suppose, is the experience of living in an area of the city which has a reputation for most forms of criminality, and where the risk of street robbery, in particular, is acute. Living with a constant fear of attack is in itself a form of victimisation and this was reported by several of our informants. Those who live in St Paul's near the centre of Bristol, or in another area of deprivation on the southern fringe of the city, have a heightened sense of risk. They cannot assume that others will treat them properly and they are surrounded by the sights and sounds of violently anti-social behaviour. Quarrels may erupt into violence on the street; a passer-by may be mugged outside your window; 'winos' may inhabit the bench outside your front-door for 24 hours a day. In such circumstances the forces of law and order can appear both distant and elusive, and the best protection is simply to keep one's mouth shut. On certain Bristol streets interpersonal violence tends to be met with practised non-intervention on the part of carefully neutral observers.

One assault victim, Julian Davies (52), explained why he felt bound to ignore the normal obligations of citizenship:

> It makes one quite tense and nervous, because if I hear these things two or three times a night, it would be silly of me to run out in the street and try to do something each time it happened . . . because I'd sooner or later get my head kicked in. At the same time, if you're lying in bed hearing it, it isn't nice.

Those who contact the police do so at some risk to themselves: another assault victim living in St Paul's described how she and others in the area would telephone the police to report violence in the street or in a nearby home but would always refuse to give their name, for fear of reprisals by their neighbours.

It is difficult to function normally under such pervasively threatening circumstances. Some of the residents of these areas whom we interviewed as assault victims were all too aware that they did not lead normal lives. Dave Knowles (41), the newspaper seller to whom reference has already been made, lives in a ground-floor flat in a particularly inhospitable and ravaged area of St Paul's. One might liken his situation to that of the 'Rule 43' prisoner except that he does not even enjoy the minimal protection afforded by prison staff. Neither a friendly neighbourhood police officer nor a prowling police van offers much protection against the potentially hostile tide of the deprived, the drunk and the violent washing against his front door. This man described his environment as 'very frightening', and we would agree.

It is important to emphasise that St Paul's contains many ordinary citizens. They comprise the great majority of its population. As Julian Davies put it to us: 'It's not like the whole area is involved in crime . . . it's just very run-down'. Nonetheless the threat of violence is always there. Davies told us that he tried to avoid places where people could be standing in the dark. He felt tense when walking in certain areas. Everyone who lives in the area suffers in this way. Davies had evidently given the matter careful thought and he repudiated the notion that the people of St Paul's entertained themselves with drugs and prostitution. He didn't think the place should be over-romanticised. There were many ordinary people and many unfortunate people who would rather be somewhere else:

There are loads of people trying to live ordinary lives.

The same may be said of residents of the massive local authority housing estate on the south-western edge of the city. Some of those whom we interviewed as assault victims were oppressed by this environment, feeling threatened both physically and psychologically by their neighbours. One couple referred to it as 'a dead end, really'. George Griffin (17), interviewed after he had been severely beaten by criminal associates, characterised it as an area of extreme tension. There was very little work, a lot of heavy drinking, and a high level of frustration. It was not unusual in local pubs for somebody to turn around and smash somebody else in the face – for nothing, as it would appear. He referred to it as 'a volatile community' in which there was tremendous hostility towards the police, expressed in baiting and taunting police officers as they drove by in their cars.

Finally we might note that it is not only those forced to live in deprived areas who suffer an increased risk of victimisation: an unfortunate piece of architectural planning may create its own hazards. A police officer, describing the narrow walkways, secluded areas and courts of a decent residential area in which Walter Drobny (32) was mugged, suggested that it had the feel of Broadwater Farm. Equally, streets which in the daytime appear unthreatening may at night become hazardous because of the drinking establishments they house, or because they are ill-lit, not much used at that time, or on the edge of high crime areas. The sense of threat afforded by this architecture is compounded by the lack of any visible police presence.

Assault victims who are themselves offenders

Another significant risk factor in relation to assault is, or appears to be, the possession of a criminal record. We say 'appears to be' because, as already acknowledged, some assaults are difficult for the outsider to penetrate so that the identity of 'victim' and 'assailant' may be in question. That said, the evidence of a relationship between criminal offending and susceptibility to assault is quite striking, and all the stronger for those assault victims who have themselves been convicted of violence. According to the author of a report on the findings of the first British Crime Survey:

> For persons reporting at least one self-reported violent offence, the likelihood of personal victimisation is 42%, or seven times the likelihood of personal victimisation for persons reporting no self-reported violence offences.

> (Gottfredson 1984: 16)

British Crime Survey data likewise suggest a close relationship between victimisation and offending, while the research conducted by Sparks *et al.* (1977) revealed a significant association between self-reported violence and the likelihood of being assaulted.

Our own hospital-based sample of ninety-two assault victims included twenty-four (26 per cent) who told us that they themselves had a criminal record, while sixteen (17 per cent) had at least one previous conviction for assault. Other offences committed by our sample of 'victims' included: shoplifting; theft; robbery with violence; and possession and dealing in drugs. With the exception of two shoplifters, all these self-confessed offenders were men. If allowance is made for the fact that some informants might be reticent about their possession of a criminal record, it can be inferred that a high proportion of assault victims are themselves convicted offenders.

The connection between a person's own offending and his or her vulnerability to assault may be explained in a variety of ways. Gottfredson suggests that:

> There is a lifestyle that for some includes high probabilities of misfortunes, victimisation and offending, due perhaps to where they

live, where they go, and with whom they associate: in other words, the social processes which produce high rates of offending in some segments of the population are also productive of high rates of victimisation.

(Gottfredson 1984: 17)

Some of our informants appeared positively to invite victimisation. For example, Darren Strudwick (89) told us that he had gone to the rescue of a stranger whom he saw being manhandled by pub bouncers. It was evident that he himself had a robust attitude to such encounters and we suspected that he may have underplayed his own involvement. Certainly he confessed to a substantial criminal record. Another youth, Kevin Pilcher (27), claimed that he was 'picked on' by bouncers in one of Bristol's more notorious city centre pubs, but he acknowledged that he himself had been imprisoned for assaulting the referee of a football match in which he had been a participant. The fact that neither of these youths shrank from aggressive confrontation may well have contributed to these incidents, even if we accept that they were not the prime movers.

The tendency for some victims to be less 'innocent' than they (or indeed we) might like to believe is particularly evident in relation to assaults perpetrated within the drugs underworld. We shall refer at some length to a youth by the name of David Freeman (4). Although clearly a 'victim' in relation to the assault which we followed, Freeman had a more daunting criminal record than any of his assailants. In particular he had committed a very nasty robbery while under the influence of drugs. The leader of the St Paul's drugs gang who tortured Freeman over a period of several hours had quite a modest criminal record by comparison. Following his decision to report his beating and abduction David Freeman was branded a 'grass': the beating which actually brought him into contact with us was relatively minor and was administered by two men who had not been involved in the first assault. This serves to emphasise how great a risk is run by people in Freeman's position when they decide to cooperate with the police. Freeman believed that his life was at risk. He had put himself in the hands of the police but he understood only too well that they were unable to protect him from the potential viciousness of the world against which he had transgressed.

Victims of violence in the drugs world typically find themselves trapped in a continuing relationship with their assailant and in this sense may be compared to victims of domestic violence. If such a person is to give evidence against an attacker, then that person will need a high degree of commitment, much courage, and as much protection as the police can afford. In fact the protection offered is almost bound to be inadequate. The officer responsible for the David Freeman case admired the way in which Freeman stood up to aggressive cross-examination at committal and at the original trial. Nonetheless he took a fairly relaxed attitude to the prospect of Freeman coming to further serious harm. There was very little he could do about that, was his view. One may infer from this that while the police purport to act on behalf of the victim, they in fact *use* the victim in furtherance of their aim of achieving a successful prosecution. This much was tacitly conceded by the officer who interviewed Timothy Paxman (6). Referring to Paxman's continuing drug addiction and his likely continued dependence on his assailant for at least part of his supply, he remarked:

> It's very sad, but they've got to help themselves, really, before we can help them.

Unfortunately there may be no real prospect of victims 'helping themselves'. The best hope, as in the Freeman case, arises where the victim manages to escape the drugs milieu. But that is not a realistic prospect for many.

Many of the inhabitants of this twilight world are known to one another and so it was that we came across 'victims' who were on friendly terms with 'assailants' in other cases which we followed. Andrew Barker (10), victim of a drunken stabbing which he himself had done much to provoke, was a close friend of one of the trio who had assaulted and abducted Freeman. We asked him where his sympathies lay in that case and they were quite clearly with the gang members. He had no time at all for Freeman whom he viewed as a 'grass'. Barker proposed to seek the advice of his solicitor following his hospitalisation with stab wounds. His assumption that he needed to secure legal advice even as a victim was perhaps not unreasonable given the murky nature of this particular incident and the fact that he was more used to being on the receiving end of police attentions. It is tempting to view incidents of this kind as relevant only to the participants and perhaps to their own closed community, rather than as criminal acts. That is certainly how they are viewed by many assailants and also, it appears, by some victims.

The victim's own role in instigating the assault

The above reflections upon the criminal careers of some assault victims lead naturally to a consideration of the extent to which victims bear some measure of responsibility for the assault which they have suffered.

The 1970s saw a developing interest in the experience and needs of crime victims, with demographic studies and other manifestations of academic and policy interest in the victim *qua* victim. For a while at least the troublesome question of whether the victim had contributed in some measure to his or her own victimisation – whether, indeed, 'victim' and 'offender' could be readily distinguished – tended to be overlooked. Subsequent 'lifestyle' studies threatened the image of the wholly innocent victim (Gottfredson 1984; Zedner 1994: 1208–10), leading to broad acceptance that the conventional stereotype is inaccurate in a great many cases. Miers refers to the dichotomy between innocent victim and blameworthy offender as 'a fundamentally inaccurate portrayal of human dynamics' (Miers 1978). We would not accept this – it may be a perfectly accurate portrayal in many instances – but we take Miers' point (see also Shapland *et al.* 1985: 188) that to ascribe to someone the status of 'victim' leaves many questions unanswered. That is why, in our own research, we took pains to try to uncover the extent of 'victim participation' in each assault. We especially wanted to gauge the impact of such victim-participation upon decisions to report and prosecute, and upon ultimate conviction and sentence. We wanted to discover, for example, whether assaults which are not reported (or which, having been reported, are not prosecuted) are those in which it is implausible to present the victim as entirely passive. This in turn might help us decide whether non-reporting should be viewed as something to worry about – a problem to be overcome – or whether, in some circumstances at least, we should regard it as appropriate and perhaps even to be encouraged.

Victim precipitation of assault has been defined as the circumstance in which 'the victim [is] the first to commence the interplay or resort to physical violence' (Wolfgang 1958: 80). In several of the cases which we followed, including some which led to a criminal trial, the victim's role remained at issue. Where the assault was reported to the police we could 'test' the victim's story against the officer's understanding of the preceding chain of events, possibly informed by the accounts of other witnesses. But in several cases we had no such yardstick. John Westcott (81) told us that he had been struck on the head while drinking in a public house – whereupon he had retaliated by hitting his attacker, this in turn provoking five or six of his attacker's friends to join in. Our 'victim' had subsequently been banned from the pub as a troublemaker. This was a typically murky tale, in which our doubts concerning the victim's story were compounded by his admitted consumption of several pints of beer. Other injured persons were even more clearly the authors of their own misfortune, having been drunk, verbally aggressive, and in at least two instances having struck the first blow. The connection between alcohol consumption and provocation is clear. Those victims who admitted having provoked their assailant (either physically or verbally) had all been drinking.

Leaving aside the cases in which victim and assailant were well known to one another, there was an element of alleged provocation (on the part of the person whom we defined as the assault victim) in thirty-two out of seventy-seven cases (42 per cent). Nonetheless we would not wish to give the impression that assault victims are, as a rule, responsible for the pains they suffer. That would be far from the truth. Even if there was some element of provocation, it was usually minimal, while the injuries inflicted were often severe and out of all proportion to any offence which might have been caused. To give one example, in the Dashwood case (3) one of the victims did do something to precipitate this assault – he attempted to 'chat up' a young girl and plonked himself in her car without any encouragement. Unfortunately he had made the grievous error of picking on the girlfriend of one of the bouncers from the pub in which he and his friends had been drinking. There was no suggestion that his behaviour was intimidatory or in any sense outrageous. Probably much more significant was the fact that these four men were an identifiable group, being strangers from the north of England. Two of them received terrible injuries, leading one to spend two days on a life-support machine and the other to suffer recurrent epileptic fits in the twelve months preceding the trial. These injuries were not in proportion to the offence of trying to chat up someone else's girlfriend.

This theme of proportionality – or rather of *disproportionate* pains suffered in response to minor provocation – was reflected in the accounts of several of the assault victims whom we interviewed. This for example was the view of Rowena Macintosh (66), a young woman who had been assaulted by a motorist who had stopped his car after she swore at him. She admitted that she made a 'V' sign and shouted various imprecations, but in her view that did not justify what followed:

> I'm quite adamant about that. I was quite justified in shouting at him – he nearly knocked us down. I just think he was in the wrong to go down the street so fast. And then for him to react like that – I just don't think I was to blame in any way whatsoever. Not at all.

Sally Chapman (60) was similarly indignant even though she admitted that she may have struck the first blow:

I did hurt him. I gave him a few punches. I was shouting, he was pushing me, I was pushing him. I can't remember, but maybe I did go for him first.

Nonetheless Chapman accepted no blame for what had happened, as was reflected in her decision to report the incident to the police. Her anger arose from what she saw as years of abuse by this man (her mother's partner). Her own admitted violence caused her no remorse because it occurred in the context of a relationship in which she felt abused.

Other victims made what they regarded as an absolute distinction between verbal aggression and physical violence. As far as they were concerned the one could never justify the other. This was a point made by women, especially, but also by some men. This was the reaction of Anthony Niblett (33) who was assaulted outside a 'gay' club from which he and his assailant had just emerged following a quarrel:

I can be quite mouthy, you know, but not *aggressively* so, that is the point.

Niblett expressed concern that some people might consider that he was to blame for the assault, having shouted out some verbal obscenity, but he comforted himself with the reflection that the violence which he had suffered was grossly disproportionate to any provocation offered.

The question of provocation also arises where victim and assailant are well known to one another and perhaps live together. In these circumstances 'provocation' may be conceived rather differently. Thirty-three of the ninety-three assaults which we followed (36 per cent) involved relationships or acquaintanceships which had given rise to difficulties in the past. In seventeen of these there had been earlier violence. Many women accepted responsibility for having provoked this or previous attacks, either by what they had said or through their own use of force. Some appeared to accept the stereotype of the 'mouthy' woman who by her verbal barbs provokes her partner to retaliate with his fists. As Alice Smythe (61) recalled:

The night that it happened I myself hadn't drunk very much. . . . I was really sharp and came back with one or two really catty remarks and that just triggered it off.

It was also clear that she herself had contributed a certain amount of physical aggression to their eighteen-month relationship. Referring to their early days together, she said:

I would hit him first. I would get *so* enraged that I would hit his face.

> And he would retaliate I suppose. But then the violence started to become habitual.

Smythe characterised this violence as 'the chemistry between us' and to that extent she accepted some responsibility for it although, being physically weaker and having better control of her drinking, as the violence became habitual she became more clearly identifiable as the victim.

But other women certainly did feel victimised. They also refused to accept that a verbal joust could justify the violence that followed. Jessie Roberts (37) told us that her partner justified his violence by reference to the 'pressure' which she imposed on him – she wanted a more committed relationship. She also conceded that . . .

> I've a fairish temper myself. It's not that I start the violence, but I won't tolerate the fact that he has other women. I will *question* him about what he's been doing.

She knew that this kind of questioning was likely to provoke violence. . . .

> but I can't be in a relationship and keep my mouth shut.

Many of these cases bring into question male definitions of what constitutes 'provocation'. If a man believes he has a right to control his partner's actions, then a great deal will be regarded as provocative. And of course many men do think this, and so regard a woman's words or deeds as a deliberate challenge to their authority. They may refer to the need to 'discipline' a woman who (whether in questioning her partner or, say, in remonstrating with a male stranger whose reckless driving has put her at risk) is seen by them to have overstepped the mark. In these circumstances the roots of the violence lie in the man's assumption of superiority and in his need to assert this in his relationships with women.

ASSAULT ARCHETYPES

We have indicated what we take to be the broad characteristics of victims and assailants and the factors contributing to risk of assault. Our own research, involving lengthy conversations with victims, enabled us to flesh out the demographic skeleton and to produce a typology of assault which differs somewhat from the categorisation employed in the 1992 British Crime Survey Report (Mayhew *et al.* 1993, chapter 6).[7] On the basis of our case studies we distinguished nine assault categories (see Figure 2.1). We conclude this chapter with a brief outline of the circumstances of each, plus some indication of the likelihood of prosecution and conviction within each archetype.

1. Assaults in pubs, clubs or dance-halls

The largest category was that of assaults in places of entertainment where alcohol is consumed. These incidents typically involve young men whose status as 'victim' or 'assailant' is likely to be contentious. The prosecution rate in respect of assaults committed on pub and club premises was low. The eighteen pub/club assaults which we followed all involved significant injury – and yet only eleven of the eighteen were reported to the police, while among those eleven cases there were just five prosecutions, all of which produced a conviction.

2. Street attacks

We distinguished between street attacks *not* having a pecuniary motive and assaults committed in the course of a robbery. A number of street attacks appeared to us to have been perpetrated simply as the result of a confrontation between rival groups of youths (e.g. between 'town' and 'gown'), while others involved an entirely random encounter between an unfortunate passer-by and a single rogue male, out of sorts with himself and all the world following a quarrel and a drinking bout (in whatever order). Victims of random attacks were not necessarily young, but all were male. Twelve of the eighteen street attacks were reported to the police but the inherent difficulties of detection in such cases is

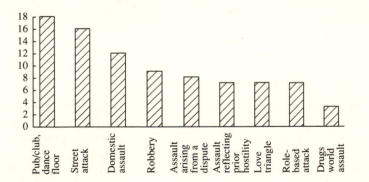

Figure 2.1 Categorisation of assaults

reflected in the fact that only four assailants were subsequently identified and prosecuted, all four being convicted.

3. Domestic assaults

Our domestic assault archetype is narrower than is sometimes reflected in the literature on the subject and certainly narrower than that employed by the police, who tend to apply the term 'domestic' to any case which involves a prior personal relationship. In only one of the twelve such cases which we identified was the assailant female. The progress of these twelve cases illustrated the considerable difficulty which domestic violence presents to the prosecuting authorities. Eight of the twelve were reported to the police. This represents a higher proportion than is thought to be typical of domestic violence cases but no doubt reflects the fact that the assaults which we followed were sufficiently serious to have prompted the victim to seek hospital treatment. In four cases out of eight the victim decided early on that she did not wish to pursue a 'complaint'; in two of the remaining four the complaint was subsequently withdrawn; and in one case the prosecution was abandoned when the victim declined to co-operate at the committal stage. There was one successful prosecution.

4. Robberies

Nine cases in our sample were 'muggings' – attacks which took place in the course of robberies. Eight of these occurred in the St Paul's area of Bristol, and we would speculate that the assailant's motive in each case was to secure money to buy drugs. Of the nine robberies in our sample *all* were reported to the police. Predictably, however, these cases posed formidable problems of detection and in the event none of the assailants was identified or prosecuted.

5. Assaults arising from a dispute

We assigned to this category assaults which were prompted by a specific disagreement between people who did *not* have a prior personal relationship. Thus we included disputes between motorists; between motorist and pedestrian; and disputes between a shopkeeper and customer. There were eight cases of this type in our sample, including several which appeared to have a racist element, although it was often difficult to determine the extent of the racial motivation. A notable feature of these assaults, as we observed them, was the high rate of reporting, investigation and prosecution. Of eight assaults, seven were reported to the police; all seven were investigated; four were prosecuted; and there were two convictions. The high rate of reporting may be accounted for by the following factors: (a) three of the incidents caused a public disturbance which brought police to the scene immediately; (b) five if not six of the victims were palpably 'innocent' and had no hesitation in seeking the assistance of the police; (c) five of the victims, perceiving themselves to have been seriously wronged, nurtured an animus against their attacker whom they wished to see punished for what had happened; and (d) in several cases the victim was seriously injured.

6. Assaults which reflect long-standing hostility between the parties

This group of seven cases included a variety of prior personal relationships, including some in which victim and assailant were distantly related or were linked by their common attachment to a third person – as where a woman was attacked by her daughter's boyfriend. One case involved a professional burglar set upon by men whom he believed nursed a grievance against him; another followed a confrontation between two young men who had been at odds since their school days. Although the injuries in these cases were generally slight the real unhappiness for the victim lay in the long-term threat which pre-dated and continued beyond the one violent incident. These seven cases were all reported, but only four gave rise to investigation by the police. This was despite the fact that, in almost every case, the assailant was readily identifiable. There were in fact three prosecutions leading to two convictions. In the three cases which went to court the history of the relationship between victim and assailant was either seriously distorted or not represented at all within the court proceedings.

7. 'Love triangles'

All the assaults within this category took place in the context of a three-cornered relationship and were motivated, broadly, by sexual jealousy. In at least three of the seven cases this appeared to have sparked off uncharacteristically violent behaviour on the part of assailants who were otherwise 'of good character'. Five of the victims were male, as were all the assailants. Two of the injured men were aged over 50; indeed, the most seriously injured victim was a man in his late sixties. Despite the fact that these incidents all arose out of a private quarrel, only one of them took place in a private dwelling and this may account for the fact that five of the seven were reported and investigated. Another factor contributing to the high reporting rate may have been the degree of injury suffered by the victims: five of the seven suffered injuries which put them in the top third of our sample in terms of severity. The five investigations led to four prosecutions and these in turn produced two convictions.

8. Role-based attacks

By 'role-based attacks' we mean assaults which are inflicted on the victim by virtue of his job (or to which he is especially vulnerable by virtue of his job). Such victims include police officers, ambulancemen, and pub landlords. Our sample of seven cases also included an amateur 'bouncer' and a university porter. With the exception of two pub landlords, the victims in this category received only slight injuries. Nonetheless a distinguishing feature of these assaults was the high rate of prosecution and conviction. Five of the seven assaults were reported to the police, and four of the assailants were prosecuted and convicted. This is a higher prosecution and conviction rate than among any of our other assault categories, although, given the numbers involved, this finding is hardly definitive.

9. Drugs world assaults

This, numerically the smallest of our case categories, involved assaults which gave rise to grave injury. These three assaults were each reported to the police and two prosecutions followed, both unsuccessful. Each of these attacks took place in the St Paul's area of Bristol. The assailants were all well known to the police as drug-dealers, some of them operating a successful rule of fear in the area. It is this rule of fear which characterises cases such as these, and it means that those victims who report violence to the police and initiate prosecution expose themselves to very great risk. The victims in these cases suffered, severally, an abduction, beating, scalding, and attempted drowning; threats with a gun followed by a savage kicking which resulted in a multiply fractured jaw; and a knife attack to the face and sustained beating with a baseball bat resulting in two broken arms. Such attacks appear to be the way in which local drug-dealers impose their authority on their customers, secure in the knowledge that this degree of intimidation affords them a measure of protection against effective prosecution.

This concludes our analysis of the circumstances of assault. In the next chapter we shall consider the impact of assault upon the victim and the way in which this bears upon the decision whether or not to go to the police. There again we shall need to pay at least as much attention to context, and relationship, as we do to the level of injury sustained.

Chapter 3

Harm and reporting

Before considering victims' response to assault, and especially their decision whether or not to go to the police, we must make some attempt to understand the effects of violence upon people of differing temperaments, in a wide variety of personal circumstances, having different kinds of relationship with their assailant. We begin with the broad generalisation that physical injury is in general of less significance than psychological harm – including the fear of further violence and a sense of humiliation at having been at someone else's mercy. Some 60 per cent of those interviewed in the course of the 1982 British Crime Survey reported that they were 'very much affected' by the violence which they had suffered. Shapland *et al.* (1985: 106) reported feelings of nervousness, anxiety, depression, lethargy and guilt on the part of the assault victims whom they interviewed. These symptoms led to behavioural changes, including avoidance of the scene of the assault and sometimes to the victim not venturing out of doors at all. A significant minority of victims suffered long-lasting fear, anxiety or depression. Shepherd *et al.* (1990b), reporting a study of forty patients attending a hospital A & E Department, observed that many assault victims displayed feelings of helplessness and bewilderment. They found it difficult to understand how the incident had developed in the way that it had. They felt 'numb', not just at being hit, but also at the fact that the attack was so unexpected and was perceived to be so unjustified. Those with no previous experience of violence were most affected. Forty per cent of assault victims had got over their distress within two weeks, but 25 per cent had still not made a full emotional recovery some six months after the attack. These researchers compared the emotional impact of assault with the distress suffered by accident victims. They reported that one week after the event the levels of anxiety and depression were similar among the two groups, but that after three months the accident victims had, in general, made a more complete recovery. They concluded that assault is more difficult to deal with than accident, often leading to a long-term loss of confidence. They also suggested that *self-blame* is more common among assault victims than it is among accident victims.

Different crime surveys produce contradictory findings concerning the impact of criminal acts (Miers 1992). This reflects the limitations of the survey method as compared with direct face-to-face interviews with the subject, but it may also reflect the nature of the offences and the victims sampled. In general, violent crime appears to have a more profound emotional impact than does non-violent crime. Thus it was concluded from the first British Crime Survey that 'crime in its most typical form does not usually have serious consequences, at least as judged by the more objective indicators of loss or injury' (Mayhew 1984: 4).[1] On the other hand, researchers who employed face-to-face interviews with known victims reported that 79 per cent of those who had suffered burglary, robbery, wounding, or snatch theft were 'very much affected' by the experience (Maguire and Corbett 1987: 42).[2]

There is doubtless a political motive in the emphasis which some victims' groups place upon the suffering of those whom they seek to represent. It has been suggested that there is some over-emphasis, if not 'sheer histrionics' in their portrayal (Gottfredson 1989: 212). Nonetheless, there is now a reputable body of evidence – from victims themselves and from specialist 'treaters' – concerning the impact of violence. Gottfredson notes the *diversity* of victims' responses, 'ranging from mild transient annoyance to profound psychological disorganisation'. This was our conclusion also, based on our monitoring of 93 assaults. Some victims appeared remarkably resilient in the face of brutal attacks. We have to consider their evidence alongside that of others who were deeply disturbed by their experience. Admittedly it is difficult, on the basis of interviews conducted within a month of the assault, to measure emotional impact in the longer term, but there was little doubt that even within that space of time some assault victims had managed to put the incident completely behind them, admitting to no lingering sense of vulnerability. There could be a variety of reasons for such apparent robustness: some victims had been intoxicated at the time of the assault and could remember little of it; others may have played some part in instigating the violence; and others may simply have possessed a phlegmatic, easy-going temperament. Many of our informants, although shaken by what had happened to them, refused to allow their lifestyle to be influenced by violence or the threat of violence.

Others were much more deeply affected. To take one example, Steven

Godden (50), despite having an apparently robust approach to physical threat, confessed that several weeks after the incident he still had difficulty sleeping and he also could not get out of the habit of staring at black men (his two assailants were black). John Enwright (39), whose injuries were likewise minor, appeared to have suffered a recurrence of a severe and disabling depression. He had attempted to return to work but on each occasion he had broken down and left early. His marital relationship had also suffered and he was having regular consultations with a psychiatrist. Rowena Macintosh (66), a young woman assaulted by a stranger, also suffered long-term distress which bore no relation to her physical injuries. She reported that the experience remained with her for some months, leading to sudden uncontrollable fits of crying. She feared for her mental stability, so disconcerted was she at her failure to control her distress in the presence of friends and colleagues. The fact that these comparatively minor assaults had such disabling consequences reminds us that whereas the law is concerned with culpability and intent, harm, especially psychological harm, is disconcertingly random.

We identified three mechanisms by which assault victims might successfully resist the loss of self-esteem which tends to flow from assault: the first of these was a determination to present oneself to the world at large as uncowed by the experience. This might be demonstrated by a willingness to face one's attacker, as in the case of Gary Atkinson (18), or by a general reluctance to fulfil the victim role – so that a refusal to report the assault to the police, for example, might be an entirely positive expression of the victim's self-reliance. This was true of Philip Harriman (15), the retired RSM assaulted in his own home by a jealous husband. He felt that in *not* reporting the attack he was showing himself to be master of his own destiny. This was a reflection of Harriman's estimation of himself as an ex-soldier, able to protect himself; in other words, his self-confidence had survived the assault.

A second aid to psychological survival was the victim's ability to say, both to himself and to the world at large, that he had been vigorous in his own defence, or in the defence of others. Several of our informants derived satisfaction from the knowledge that they had struck some effective blows, or at least had acted bravely. Steven Clutton (8) received extremely serious injuries (fractured skull, broken jaw and lost teeth) for which he was still receiving treatment when interviewed five months after the assault. But his actions at the time in going back to protect his friend, thereby leading to his own far more serious injuries, enabled him to recall the incident with pride. The fact that he had become a hero to his friends gave him something positive to hold on to.

The opposite was the case with Sean Bradenham (62), the young man who was injured at a university function where he was employed in the role of amateur 'bouncer'. He suffered minor physical injury (a broken nose), but there was a severe blow to his ego because having been employed to maintain order he had been worsted by a single blow.

A third device for maintaining self-esteem is to convert the whole incident into something of a party-piece. In the case of Donald Burke (55), the man assaulted in the toilets of Bristol Royal Infirmary, the sheer absurdity of what had happened (perhaps coupled with the fact that his injuries were not serious), made for an entertaining story which he and his family clearly enjoyed telling. A parallel case was the un-provoked attack on Louise Duke (69) and her friend: they were not seriously threatened, their attacker was unknown to them, and their subsequent contact with the police was something of an adventure. Unfortunately this was not true of most of the assaults which we followed. The incidents were too private, revealed the victim in too unflattering a light, or were too painful in their effects, to be transformed into enter-tainment.

There were two circumstances in particular which tended to ag-gravate victims' loss of self-esteem. The first of these was a feeling on the victim's part that he or she bore some responsibility for the events leading up to the assault. The question of responsibility, and consequent guilt, raises much broader questions than are reflected in Wolfgang's definition of 'the victim being the first to commence the interplay or resort to physical violence' (Wolfgang 1958): it is a question of the person's moral identity. Some victims were rendered more anxious and depressed because they felt that they themselves had caused the attack, but that did not mean that an independent observer would have judged them 'responsible' in any meaningful sense. Gerald Abbott (31), knocked down and kicked in the head by a drunken (or drugged) youth whose attention he had had the misfortune to catch, told us:

> I'm dwelling on it all the time . . . I keep blaming myself for getting involved in that situation.

Alex Thomas (75), who was assaulted when he interrupted a youth engaged in an act of vandalism, still felt disturbed by his part in the incident when we spoke to him four weeks later:

> There's an element of shame in the whole thing in that I spoilt a good evening with friends. I went a little too far and provoked a physical attack.

Both these men (the first a retired policeman whose sense of responsibility was compounded by his feeling that as a 'professional' he should have been able to look after himself) displayed remorse which others, whose responsibility appeared to us far greater, did not share. *We* might think that Abbott and Thomas were being over-scrupulous, but the important point is that the impact of assault depends in part upon the victim's personal identity; if the victim is inclined towards self-blame for any misfortune, then the psychological burden he or she carries is likely to be that much greater.

The other factor which we noted as aggravating the emotional impact of assault was the victim's having to be off work for any length of time. This fate befell Patrick Mangan (13) and Timothy Cooper (20), the two pub landlords who figured in our sample – one because he had suffered a broken knee-cap and the other because tendons in his hand had been damaged. Both these men were very upset at the effect of their injuries upon their daily lives. They were concerned that they could no longer work behind the bar, concerned about the effect on their business, and worried also by the increased burden which had to be borne by their wives. The depression which they suffered seemed to arise from the loss of their work effectiveness, rather than from any trauma occasioned by the assault.

TOLERANCE OF VIOLENCE

Just as some people are more prepared than others to *use* violence, it can be inferred that there are very great differences in people's tolerance of violence employed by others. Broadly speaking, those victims of assault for whom physical violence was not the norm tended to be more shocked by their victimisation than were those who inhabited a world in which it was normal to settle arguments by recourse to boots and fists. Many of the assault victims whom we interviewed admitted that they were themselves violent on occasion. Gary Atkinson (18), for example, told us that when younger he had had a violent temper. Even now . . . 'if a friend is in trouble, I'll always help'. So Gary had been involved in several fights, including some in the pub where he suffered such a brutal beating. Similarly, Jonathan Dowson (48), a Hell's Angel (as he described himself) who had been assaulted with a snooker cue, appeared unaffected by the incident beyond retaining a sense that he and his adversary still had unfinished business to attend to. The fact that he was only slightly injured, coupled with his membership of a community in which violence is habitual, at least in dress, discipline and imagination, caused him to perceive the assault as but a minor matter.

Certain individuals, by the nature of their work, are exposed to violence. A police officer or ambulance driver may be able to accept an assault as part of the job. Jonathan Musgrove (45), a police officer injured off-duty, said that he would have felt much *less* upset had the attack occurred while at work. This sentiment was consistent with the views expressed by those victims who had been assaulted 'in role': the fact that the violence had not been directed against the victim in a personal capacity served to diminish the anger and sense of threat experienced. Ronald Pratt (28), a police officer who had his nose broken in the course of making an arrest, was able to refer to it as 'part of the job'. He denied any sense of outrage (although he was very upset that his assailant was given only a suspended prison sentence):

> I don't take it personally; he wasn't hitting me because I'm Ronald Pratt; he was hitting me because I was a policeman and I was in his way of escape – it's just one of those things.

Where violence is not reported this may be because it has little impact upon the victim or upon observers. However, one should not *assume* tolerance of violence, even on the part of those who experience quite a lot of it. We know, for example, that it is the norm for students who suffer injuries in Bristol University Students' Union not to report the matter to the police. The reasons for this might include a wish to avoid the inconvenience associated with reporting; a preference for maintaining tolerable relations within that community; a dislike of the police; a sense of contributory responsibility – in fact most of the reasons for non-reporting which we encountered. But it would be unwise to conclude from this that students are in general 'tolerant of violence'. The same applies to those at the other end of the social scale who suffer habitual violence because of their drunkenness or homelessness. Some of our most deprived informants were oppressed by all the circumstances of their lives: they did not so much tolerate violence as feel bound to endure it.

ASSAULTS IN A 'DOMESTIC' CONTEXT

Our informants included twelve women who had been attacked by the man with whom they lived or with whom they were involved; eight had subsequently broken off the relationship, while the remainder appeared content to continue in it, or rather, in some instances, to continue it on revised terms. It was sometimes difficult to be sure whether those women who expressed a firm intention in either direction would in fact adhere to it.

Where a woman had been habitually victimised by her partner it was not always the most serious attack which prompted her to go to the police: the intervention of another family member might lead to police involvement which in turn might prompt a break in the relationship. But in some cases the woman appeared to expect so little from the relationship that she was prepared to accept the violence: Linda Hutt (34) had been involved with her assailant for 21 years, the relationship having been violent from the start. After the first five years, when Linda's child was born, she and her partner lived apart although he continued to come to her council flat casually, as and when he wanted, staying for days at a time. We encountered Linda in hospital with a damaged tendon sustained when this man had thrown a glass at her in the course of an argument. It appeared that she still valued his companionship, when he chose to give it her. She had not reported this latest incident to the police.

At the same time we should recognise that a failure to report domestic assault to the police does not necessarily denote passivity. Some women, whether because of their intelligence, their robust temperament, or their relative independence (in terms of earning power, accommodation, and childlessness) do not see themselves as victims. Jane Bond (68), who made a 999 call following a fight with her boyfriend, acknowledged that she was herself violent on occasion and claimed that some of her female friends behaved similarly:

> There are a lot of violent relationships. I think it's because women are so much more stronger now and want their rights and want an equal partnership and feel that they can express themselves. I think women are much more willing to express themselves in a violent way now. [Pause] A lot of it, you think . . . I can hit him, he can't hit *me*.

Jane had by her own account instigated this latest violent episode. She was acting, according to her own perception, from a position of strength, with her boyfriend being the real 'victim'. She also regarded this eruption of violence as marking a turning point in their relationship: she and her boyfriend were subsequently reconciled and Jane believed that the violence had had a therapeutic effect.

This idea that assault acts as a kind of watershed in an intimate relationship is worthy of a little more development. It is first necessary to acknowledge that in cases where the woman told us that she and her partner were now 'operating on a new basis' – or similar term – we had no way of knowing whether these resolutions would be sustained. Ours was a snapshot view. In many instances we were conscious of the fragility of the relationship and of the brittleness of some of the personalities involved. One typical scenario was where one partner (or both) had resolved to stop drinking, or to drink less than hitherto. Alice Smythe (61) was attending Al-Anon[3] where she believed she had learned a workable technique for dealing with her partner's drink-induced violence. His evident instability (he had attempted suicide a few months before this assault and been recommended for psychiatric treatment, which he did not take up) made it harder for her to break with him, although it appeared that she had never seriously considered this. Although there was some evidence, therefore, that this particular attack had been a turning point in the relationship between this couple, there was also a sense that the old momentum of violence might reassert itself. Or as Smythe put it to us at the end of our interview:

I'm living from day to day. . . . I dread it all starting again.

That of course does suggest something of the powerless victim, rather than the empowered captain of her fate which was how women such as Jane Bond presented themselves.[4]

Another kind of watershed is the circumstance where an assault prompts the woman finally to terminate a long-running but fundamentally unsatisfactory relationship. Here again the same caveat applies: even where the victim presented what had happened to her as some kind of turning-point in her life, we could not be certain that her resolution would be sustained. Many of these relationships were marked by previous bouts of violence, and previous separations. Admittedly we were sometimes told that the incident which we were following had been the most severe, or had had the most dramatic repercussions – had been, in other words, a real turning-point. The women who claimed that this really was 'the end' tended to be the ones who had at least minimal security and support from other sources – usually from other members of their family. This bears on one of the themes which we shall be developing in this book: that the fleeting intervention of police and courts can never be sufficient in itself to free a woman from dependence upon perhaps the only source of support and companionship which she knows and, in some limited sense, can rely on.

REPORTING

Having considered, albeit briefly, the impact of assault upon the victim, we now turn to a consideration of the first stage of the criminalisation process, this being the victim's decision whether or not to report the assault to the police. It is possible to view the criminal justice process as a series of key decision-making points, each of course having some relationship to the others. *Early* decisions (at least if closing off the prosecution option) may be regarded as more powerful than later ones (Hindelang and Gottfredson 1976: 57). The decision whether or not to report an assault to the police is in this sense the most crucial: the assault victim in effect exercises a power of veto over the prosecution process. The police, as is well known, do not for the most part stumble upon or in any sense 'discover' crime: criminal offences become known to them because they are reported by members of the public – most commonly, by the victim.[5]

It can be assumed that the increased rate of recorded assault, which we reported in Chapter 1, reflects greater public sensitivity towards interpersonal violence as well as, perhaps, a greater confidence in the willingness of the police and 'authority' generally to take such offences seriously. Hood, for example, considers the argument that a greater readiness to report violent crime reflects an increased sensitivity to anti-social behaviour rather than a rise in violence *per se* (Hood and Sparks 1970: 43), and cites Biderman's observation that 'year to year increases in crime rates may be more indicative of social progress than social decay' (Biderman 1966). Of course it could be a combination of progress *and* decay, but the point we wish to make here is that a greater willingness to report violence – to *complain* about it – can be interpreted positively as marking a refusal to submit to such behaviour. It also, presumably, reflects some belief in the state's willingness to protect assault victims and punish those who have been violent towards them. The police for their part, provided they take the victim seriously, can reinforce this sense that violence will not be tolerated. As Hough and Mayhew put it (1985: 54), recording crime is a symbolic function of the police . . . 'formally marking the boundary between acceptable and criminal behaviour and the legitimacy of the victim's sense of grievance'.

The question of what proportion of assaults is reported to the police is not easy to answer, depending as it does upon one's definition both of 'reporting' and of 'assault'. Attempts have been made, based upon survey data, one example being the victimisation surveys conducted by the National Crime Survey Panel in the USA. Their findings indicated a

56 per cent rate of non-reporting for assaults, the same proportion as for rapes (Hindelang *et al*. 1975). The 1992 British Crime Survey indicated that 48 per cent of woundings and 26 per cent of common assaults were reported to the police (Mayhew *et al*. 1993: 15). Our own research evidence is of value here because it taught us the remarkable indeterminacy of the 'reporting' concept. This theme will be developed further in succeeding chapters, but the nub of the issue is the operational distinction which the police maintain between 'reporting' and 'complaining' – a distinction which is, unsurprisingly, unclear to many assault victims. This is not simply a matter of the police declining to record an offence reported to them (in police argot, 'cuffing' the incident); 'making a complaint' is a police term of art which means *you are prepared to take this all the way to court and, if necessary, to give evidence*. Thus we find, in relation to the ninety-three assaults whose progress we monitored, that seventy-five (81 per cent) were reported to the police – either by the victim (forty-one cases) or by a third party (thirty-four cases) – but in only forty-seven of these cases (63 per cent) did the victim make a formal statement. In the other twenty-eight cases the assault was not recorded or else there was deemed to be 'no complaint'.

Demographic variables associated with reporting

One factor which appears to have some bearing upon whether offences (not only of assault) are reported to the police is the age of the victim. The 1984 British Crime Survey found that victims aged under 26 were less likely to report all but the most serious crimes (Hough and Mayhew 1985: 25). Suggested reasons were: younger victims had less favourable attitudes towards the police; the crimes suffered by young people tended to be different; and there was less likelihood of younger victims having insurance cover. Needless to say, only the first of these bears upon the reporting of assault. The 1984 British Crime Survey also found that *the better educated* were more likely to report offences to the police (again, this is in relationship to crime in general, not specifically to assault) (*ibid*.: 25). This finding has been replicated in the USA (Gottfredson and Hindelang, 1979). And finally we may note the observation by Schneider (1976: 146) that the decision to report is influenced by the victim's degree of integration or involvement in their local community. Victims were less likely to report if they "understood local issues".

These data, being derived from reporting rates in respect of all types of crime, tell us little about reporting patterns in respect of assault. Indeed, Sparks *et al*. (1977: 120) conclude that it is best to ignore these demographic 'findings', if such they be, since victim decisions to report an offence are incident specific. That may be true, but it is nonetheless possible, by focusing upon specific categories of assault, to come up with useful generalisations. One impressive piece of work of this type is the study of the relationship between *race* and reporting conducted by Shah and Pease (1992). These researchers found that assaults committed by non-whites were more likely to be reported, but that this applied particularly to assaults where there was no injury. In addition, black offenders in groups were more likely to be reported than were white offenders operating as a group. The authors conclude that race (which in the case of assailants means *perceived* race) is a factor in the decision not to report, over and above other offence variables: there is in general a lower reporting threshold when the offender is non-white; race factors cannot be reduced to offence factors. But while there does appear to be discrimination the researchers make it clear that this discrimination operates in a complex way.

The relationship between offence seriousness and reporting

Despite the information now available to suggest that willingness to report, as well as susceptibility to assault in the first place, is to some extent a function of the victim's age, sex and race, there appears to be a general consensus, arrived at on the basis of survey data, that victims' perception of *seriousness* is the main factor determining whether or not they go to the police. This was a finding of all the British Crime Surveys (Hough and Mayhew 1985: 19; Mayhew *et al.* 1989: 24; Mayhew *et al.* 1993: 26): the main reason for non-reporting, in relation to all criminal offences, was the victim's perception that what had happened to him or her was relatively trivial. In the 1992 British Crime Survey 55 per cent of 'non-reporting' victims gave this as their reason for taking matters no further. Gottfredson and Hindelang (1979) reported, on the basis of the National Crime Survey data in the USA, that 'by far the strongest correlate of the decision to call the police was the seriousness of the crime experienced by the victim'. They concluded that 'judging by victimization surveys, demographic and social characteristics of victims appear to play little role in the decision to call the police'.

It seems to us that there is something inherently unsatisfactory about adopting seriousness *as defined by the victim* as a measure and then relating this to reporting behaviour.[6] We shall argue on the basis of our own research evidence that this 'finding' is at best banal, or platitudinous, and at worst thoroughly misleading. Of course it is true that victims' perceptions that they have suffered only moderate harm is a factor in non-reporting, but the important thing to understand is that while triviality, or perception of triviality, may deter reporting, *seriousness of injury is not in itself sufficient to ensure that an assault is reported*. Seriousness can be outweighed by other factors. What is more, some very serious assaults are reported in a matter which makes it highly unlikely that the police will pursue an investigation. One example concerns Gary Atkinson (18), the young man beaten up in a pub toilet. Atkinson did indeed attend a police station but his ambivalence was apparent in that, for reasons connected with the character of his assailant and the fact that he was bound to encounter him again, he chose not to give his name to the police. We observed many other cases which confirmed that while 'seriousness' is important, it is far from overriding (Clarkson *et al.*, 1994).

Reasons why assault victims go to the police

It would be a mistake to imagine that most assaults are reported to the police. Failure to report should not be regarded as aberrant: it is the norm. We shall now, with the aid of our own research findings, consider reasons *for* reporting. First there is the victim's sense of social responsibility. According to the 1984 British Crime Survey, 33 per cent of all crime victims referred to a sense of obligation as underpinning their decision to go to the police (Hough and Mayhew 1985: 18). To report the offence was 'the right thing to do' (Shapland *et al.* 1985: 15). Some of our informants likewise expressed this sense of social obligation, perhaps referring to the risk to others, or suggesting that to report crime as a matter of routine might increase the level of policing. The inconvenience of reporting, which might be considerable, was outweighed by the person's sense of obligation to his or her fellow citizens. As Robert James (63) put it to us:

> A lot of people said there's no point, they won't be able to do anything. I thought, if it happened again next week and somebody got killed, then I wouldn't be able to live with myself if I hadn't reported it . . . and I could have quite easily been very badly hurt or killed.

Few of those who reported their assault appeared to have taken into consideration the possibility of their being called upon as a witness. One who had done so was Anthony Niblett (33), whose job as a social worker brought him into contact with children appearing before the courts in child abuse cases. He thought that he should pursue the case against his assailant, however unpleasant the consequences for himself, because: 'I think I have an obligation to society . . . a duty if you like.'

Another motive for reporting assault, particularly in circumstances where victim and assailant were known to one another, was the victim's wish to see her assailant confronted with his behaviour in a public forum. For many victims it is this, rather than anticipation of the court's sentence, which persuades them that they ought to go to the police. Public recognition that the assault had taken place would, it was hoped, vindicate the victim and at the same time have some impact upon her assailant. Josephine Macdonald (51), attacked by her ex-boyfriend, no longer viewed him as a potential threat *to her*; but she was concerned that he be made to recognise that what he had done was wrong:

> I think I'm not really hopeful that the court can really *do* anything. I don't think they can impose any really severe penalty and I'm not sure I'd want them to if they could, but I feel that I'm bothering to take the case to court, even given that it might perhaps bring more trouble later, simply that the nature of the man's mind might be such that . . . [pause] he might be inclined to forget that he'd done a thing like that. And even if they're only going to give him some sort of token fine I felt just that it will reinforce that he had done such a thing and that it was assault.

Rowena Macintosh (66) was another who expressed the hope that criminal prosecution would confront her assailant with his own behaviour. She was not interested, she said, in revenge:

> I just don't see that it would do any good. As far as I'm concerned I don't want to inflict punishment on the guy at all. Not in the slightest. But I'd like him to be made aware of what he's done.

This same wish to see their assailant experience a public calling to account was expressed by many other assault victims whom we interviewed. Formal punishment was incidental; they wanted a public statement. It is an unfortunate fact, to which we shall return, that a finding of guilt and the passing of sentence does not necessarily bring with it any convincing or resounding public message. Indeed, the muddled, low key nature of most magistrates' courts, coupled with the demeanour of the defendant (even more so, of the *defendants*, where jointly charged) can undermine any hoped-for impression of seriousness. If the victim is seeking effective public condemnation of the defendant, she is likely to be disappointed.

A third reason why assault victims choose to go to the police is that, fearing further attacks, they want to find some way of controlling their assailants' future behaviour. William Kenny (43), hit over the head with a brick by someone at whose hands he had suffered a previous assault, reported the second incident because he wanted to see his assailant deterred from further violence:

> If it had been a slap, where I'd suffered a cut lip, I probably wouldn't have bothered. But this was serious. What worried me more than anything is, if I leave it and I'm walking down the High Street in a year or two years' time, and he's already hit me with a brick, what's he gonna do the next time? . . . It might put him in line a bit. At least he'll have a record. Then, if he continued to hit people, they're gonna deal with him in a more serious manner aren't they?

In this case the offender was successfully prosecuted, but it is quite common for victims who go to the police for reasons of their own protection not to receive the help which they think they need. They may be very vulnerable people who, nonetheless, do not attract police sympathy – perhaps because they are held to be of little value in the currency of the courts. Mushtak Iqbal (87) was a case in point. Iqbal had made several complaints to the police, also informing them of minor criminal infractions which he had observed, such as cars being parked on double yellow lines or without road tax. He could not understand the indifference with which these reports had been greeted. This latest incident involved a punch in the chest (truly, a common assault) which the police were not disposed to act upon. The man who hit Iqbal continues to live in the neighbourhood and is often within shouting distance. Iqbal wanted protection: it was evident to him that his assailant had not been deterred. At the time of our contact with him he was still seeking some manifestation of police authority. He did not necessarily want his tormentor arrested: he just wanted his trouble to end. The lack of any effective police response meant that he was not sure that it *had* ended.

Other assault victims, although unsatisfactory to varying degrees from the police perspective, were more fortunate. Alison Browne (65), a middle-aged woman who acknowledged her own drink problem, had been assaulted by her son. She went to the police when further violence threatened, principally to protect herself from a second beating. She was gratified by their response. She showed the officer her bruises and said that she was afraid to stay in her own home that night. The officer had apparently responded to the effect: 'I know you're not (staying in the house).' This phrase, 'I know you're not', was repeated to the researcher several times, with evident satisfaction, by Browne. She had never had any intention of triggering a criminal prosecution – a fact made clear to the officer. In this case it was probably helpful to have the police arrive to defuse the situation in the Browne home and convey to the son that violence against his mother was not to be tolerated, no matter that he may have been provoked by her abuse and drunkenness. The violence in this household was probably deep-rooted in that it arose from the heavy drinking of both mother and son, and from the frustrations of their intimacy. Nonetheless the fact that on this occasion Browne received a sympathetic and practically useful response was very important to her. This was despite the fact that there was never any prospect of a court being involved.

Despite the occasional success story, it was more common to find the police *failing* to give vulnerable assault victims the protection which they thought they needed. Dave Knowles (41) exemplified this problem. Knowles had been assaulted many times and was well known at his local police station. He regarded the police as his friends (although this had not prevented him from bringing the occasional complaint against them). He trusted them to investigate his allegations of assault, or of robbery (Knowles lived in a difficult area) and on the whole they had done so. At least one of Knowles' complaints had led to criminal prosecution. Knowles is not, however, a satisfactory complainant from the police point of view. He is confused; he drinks; he embellishes stories even if he does not completely make them up; he is occasionally violent himself; he reports *too many* crimes. In this instance Knowles reported that he had been 'mugged' while delivering newspapers, being robbed of over £100, but on this occasion, as we believe on others, no crime report was made out. As far as the official record was concerned, Knowles had not been assaulted. It was plain to us that he had indeed suffered violence, although at whose hand, and in what circumstances, we would not like to say.

Another possible motive for reporting assault is the victim's wish to secure financial compensation – either from the assailant as ordered by the court, or from the state through the Criminal Injuries Compensation Board. Police officers whom we interviewed sometimes expressed a certain scepticism with regard to victims' motives in reporting violent crime: they suspected that a desire to secure an award from the CICB might prompt an 'unworthy' victim to complain. On the other hand it has been observed that 'it does not appear to be the case that the provision of financial reparation (from whatever source) is a significant factor in the reporting of offences against the person' (Miers 1976). Our evidence supports this: we came across only one case in which we noted that a financial motive lay behind the victim's decision – that of George Griffin (17), who went to the police some weeks after he had been assaulted when he learned of the existence of the CICB. (In fact the CICB turned him down on the grounds of (a) his criminal record and (b) the length of time taken to report the matter.)

For the most part our informants made no reference to the possibility of their securing compensation. We need not infer from this that they would have turned it down if offered: it may rather be that they did not believe they were likely to get it – either from the CICB or from their assailant. Even someone who has only the most passing acquaintance with the criminal courts is likely to have absorbed the message that they do not offer much in the way of compensation to victims. Most of our informants, when asked what they considered would be an appropriate punishment for their attacker, appeared content with the idea of a fine. They did not by and large suggest that their attacker should also pay compensation. It seemed that even those who most determinedly sought prosecution did not anticipate that this would lead to financial recompense. Nor, for the most part, did they have a view of justice which incorporated this idea. It was not what they expected. The CICB of course was set up with the express purpose of providing financial compensation for assault victims, but it has a comparatively low profile and we found that most of our informants had either not heard of it or did not believe that their injuries were serious enough for them to qualify.

Reasons for not reporting

We now turn to reasons for *not* reporting assault and these, as will soon become apparent, are more numerous and in many instances more powerful than those factors which incline victims to go to the police. First we consider victims' perceptions of the *detectability* of the offence. It goes almost without saying that one reason why assault victims may choose not to report the incident is that they do not know the identity of their assailant(s) and therefore see no prospect of the crime being detected (Hough and Mayhew 1985: 65). Assault victims seem to have rather low expectations of the police: they understand only too well that the police do not behave in the manner or rejoice in the success rate of Hercule Poirot or Inspector Morse – or at least, they do not behave like this in relation to common-or-garden assault. In so far as our informants understood this, their perceptions were in accord with academic research findings concerning police reliance upon members of the public to 'detect' crime. As one observed:

> There's not a lot of point going to the police because I don't know who did it.

Several of the victims whom we interviewed had no need to rely upon fictional portrayals of the police – they had their own experience to go on. This need not have turned them against the police, or rendered them cynical, but it tended to ensure that they did not have unreasonable expectations. As Edward Billingston (57) observed:

> There didn't seem any point. I didn't get any clear view of the person, to give a good description. No one else saw it. What could they do? They wouldn't be interested. I know from past experience that . . . small assaults like that, they don't seem to be interested in following them up. I suppose the manpower . . . it just doesn't seem worth it.

As we shall demonstrate, victims are amply justified in having these low expectations of the police in circumstances where they themselves cannot assist in the identification of their assailant.

A second, more positive reason for non-reporting is the assault victim's refusal to accept a 'victim' identity: some people regard a decision to go to the police as tantamount to a request for help which in their case they do not need. Although there is a tendency to view non-reporting as negative – a symptom of the victim's oppression – there are instances where non-reporting bears a positive construction. For example, Bob Deane (85) expressed wry amusement at his assailant's threats:

> He said he was from a peace convoy and he was going to get the rest of the peace convoy to come up and sort me out at a later date and this, that, and the other. Which goes over the top of my head.

He did not feel personal animus against his attacker. The incident was seen as role-based, between steward and customer.

This same positive construction may, on occasion, be applied to non-reporting by victims of 'domestic' assault, or by male protagonists in a 'love triangle'. Philip Harriman (15) did not see himself as requiring the support of the law. He was able to explain what had happened as a private event in which his own position, even though he had been seriously injured, was more powerful (and more enviable) than that of his assailant. Some assault victims do not lack power in relation to their assailant, and this is true even of domestic assault. Some women who are assaulted by their partners perceive what has been done to them as their fault (Mayhew *et al.* 1993: 130), but others, we believe, accept partial responsibility not from a position of weakness but as a way of demonstrating their pride and independence. As Alice Smythe (61) put it: 'I don't *feel* as if I'm a victim.' Her decision not to involve the police should be viewed in this light.

Another group of victims who chose not to report assaults were physically confident young men assaulted in a pub or nightclub by a stranger. In each case they intended to continue frequenting such places, believing that they could look after themselves. It was not only because they felt that there was no realistic chance of detection that they did not go to the police; they exhibited a degree of self-confidence and self-reliance which meant that they were reluctant to accept the 'victim' label. They did not consider that they needed police assistance in relation to what were, for them, relatively minor incidents. It is perhaps paradoxical that people like this who are, broadly speaking, unimpaired by the assault which they have suffered and who would therefore make excellent 'complainants' from the point of view of the police tend to be the ones who see no need for such involvement. Perhaps, after all, that is appropriate: we are talking here of relatively minor incidents, in which case a few retaliatory blows struck at the time may offer more tangible satisfaction than would engagement in the criminal justice enterprise.

Fear of reprisals and the decision to report

In the 1988 British Crime Survey fear of reprisals was given as a reason for non-reporting in 2 per cent of common assaults, in 3 per cent of other assaults, and in 5 per cent of woundings (Mayhew *et al.* 1989: 74). The US National Crime Survey Panel found that 4 per cent of victims gave fear of reprisals as their reason for not reporting an assault, although the proportion doubled in relation to more serious cases (Hindelang *et al.* 1975). It is our contention that survey data significantly under-represents the degree to which *assault victims*, in particular, are deterred from going to the police through fear. Fear of reprisals was acknowledged by some 14 per cent of the victims whom we interviewed. It was especially prominent where victim and assailant had an on-going relationship – whether as partners, family members, *habitués* of a common social environment such as a pub, or as members of the drugs underworld. In each of these disparate circumstances it was held that neither the police nor the courts would be able to prevent further attacks were the assailant so minded. For example, Gary Atkinson (18), knew his assailant well and was thoroughly intimidated by him. He had asked the police whether, if he chose to identify this man, he would be granted bail. The police indicated that he well might – and that was enough for Atkinson. As he said to us:

> At the very least I'd be threatened – if not by him, then by other people. I don't think it would get to court very smoothly, put it that way. I'd be intimidated – at the *least* intimidated. It's not fear of what he would do to me – because he can't do much more in all honesty – but I don't particularly want another hiding like this one. So common sense prevails.

The most dramatic examples of non-reporting by reason of intimidation were in relation to assaults perpetrated within the drugs underworld. Each of these was serious – and the police took them seriously – but each prosecution failed because the victim was afraid to go through with the process. These cases revealed the inadequacy of the protection available to assault victims who inhabit this milieu. Serious assault is a grim business at the best of times, but there is all the difference in the world between, say, a blow struck in the course of a dispute between two motorists and the assault suffered by Timothy Paxman (6). In the one case, where there is no on-going relationship marked by power imbalance between victim and assailant, the victim's course of action is straightforward – report the matter to the police and assist in any way possible with the prosecution process. But where there is an on-going power relationship – as in 'domestic' violence, or where a drug baron rules his particular fiefdom by means of his ruthless commitment to violence – there may be no effective remedy. The police may be enthusiastic, certainly where there is a good chance of successful prosecution, but if the victim is reluctant to co-operate, perhaps because intimidated (or, in the case of Paxman, in fear of his life) then the police take the matter no further. So there is a great difference between the degree of victimisation suffered by different assault victims. The striking common element in drugs world assaults and domestic violence is the extent to which the focus upon prosecution fails to meet the victim's need for security in the future. This of course is counter-productive to the extent that victims in this position are inadequately supported in their fragile commitment to the prosecution effort.

Victim attitude and lifestyle

The extent of unreported violence among those who are marginalised – the homeless and those who spend much of their lives on the streets, often under the influence of drink or drugs – we judge to be considerable. For such victims (who may as often be themselves offenders) reporting is unlikely to present itself as an attractive option. A generally oppressed lifestyle, coupled perhaps with a hostile attitude to the forces of law and order, can lead to a perception that violence is inescapable. As we have previously emphasised, this is not to be confused with a so-called 'tolerance of violence'. The factors which contribute to non-reporting are too many and too complex to allow such a blanket classification. Those who regularly suffer violence may not tolerate it, but rather be unable to avoid it or seek a remedy for it. Even those victims of assault whose lives are as described may, on occasion, have recourse to the police in an attempt to secure protection and vindication. In that case they are less likely than the rest of us to receive it. Their damaged status renders them of little value in the currency of the courts. We did encounter one woman, Sally Chapman (60 and 88), who admitted to having herself been violent in the past and who was also, by her own account, a drinker, a lesbian, and resident of St Paul's. She had nonetheless reported these incidents to the police with the intention of securing public condemnation of her assailants' behaviour. But she faced formidable obstacles, not least her own lack of innocence as reflected in her drinking and her violence. Criminal proceedings in respect of the two assaults on Ms Chapman were aborted by the police and the CPS respectively.

There were also young men among our sample who regarded the use of fists and feet as an acceptable way of settling an argument and who did not, therefore, look to the police for protection: Jonathan Dowson (48), while insisting that he was 'not a violent man', belonged to a 'biker' culture which conceived of at least some violent acts as expressions of discipline. No biker, said Dowson, would report an assault to the police; any infringement of their own code would be dealt with internally. Non-reporting in these circumstances might suggest that the victim was subject to an alternative justice system, one characterised by 'acceptable' violence.

It is unsurprising that those who live on the margins of criminality are less likely than the supposedly upright citizen to seek police assistance when they are assaulted. George Griffin (17) told us that he would not dream of identifying his assailant to the police

because I'm not a grass . . . I would lose my credibility.

On occasion we observed serious assaults on 'marginal' figures being reported by third parties: such cases invariably posed problems for the police (and, subsequently, for the CPS) because, typically, the victim was ambivalent about engaging in the justice process. Andrew Barker (10) was one such: he had suffered a very serious assault – six stab wounds in the chest, leading to a collapsed lung. One might have thought that there would be no question about his cooperating with the prosecution of his (known) assailant, but in fact Barker was ambivalent about this. He may have been one assault victim for whom the option of 'private justice' (see below) was a realistic prospect, although we understand that in the end the affair was effectively 'buried' by the two men and their respective supporters. In the circumstances Barker's failure to turn up to give evidence at his assailant's trial for GBH was not unexpected, the officer in the case having earlier expressed surprise at Barker's willingness to cooperate:

> Normally people of that ilk tend to bury their own dead . . . so I'm surprised it's being pursued . . . by him.

Our research sample included at least a dozen assault victims whose 'innocence' was very much in question. Some were drug addicts; some had criminal records in relation to other matters; some were suspected by the police of having been less than frank in their accounts of what brought them to the area where they had been assaulted – as for example Steven Godden (50), the middle-class businessman complete with laptop computer who claimed that he had lost his way while driving through St Paul's but whom the police suspected of having been in search of a prostitute. These victims presented, or were seen to present, a problem for the police. It was anticipated that they would, for one reason or another, prove unsatisfactory complainants. Were the case to get as far as a court they were likely not to attend, or else to prove unsatisfactory witnesses – or so the police evidently thought. As one officer explained, referring to the St Paul's area of the city:

> In that area down there there's a lot of prostitution, and people go in, get assaulted, won't report it because they're embarrassed and all that. It causes immense problems with the investigation, because if you're not told the truth by the aggrieved person on the day, you ain't gonna get to the truth now.

Having observed the trial process, it is not difficult to understand why some victims would not want an account of their movements revealed to the world at large. This is a problem with a great many victims – they are not innocent enough. They are not innocent enough to convince the police of the truth of their story, or to convince them that they are

prepared to see the prosecution through; and if those hurdles are sur-
mounted they may still not be innocent enough to convince a court.
Some of our informants, through their previous experience of the police,
had come to understand this. They believed, in other words, that they
had forfeited their right to police protection and to the remedies which
the law provides. A relatively trivial example is provided by Edward
Billingston (57), who admitted to us that he had been drunk at the time
he was assaulted. Not only did Billingston judge that his case would not
be detectable; he also doubted whether the police would be committed
to detecting it. This was based partly on his experience of the police in
relation to an earlier assault, and partly upon his understanding of the
police attitude (and that of hospital staff) towards drinkers:

> You haven't been to a church social if you're brought in at 4 o'clock
> in the morning, have you? You're *bound* to have been out drinking.
> Some people do get violent when they've been drinking, I suppose.
> And therefore, when you come in with a bloody nose and you've
> been drinking, they assume you've provoked somebody or, if you've
> been involved in a fight, you're to blame as much as they are. And I
> think the police think that as well: if you've been drinking, you're
> automatically not worth bothering about. You've brought it on yourself.

It was salutary to note how many people appear to accept that they have
moved beyond the law's protection. To appeal to authority in the face of
violence is not an option as far as they personally are concerned.

Provocation, blameworthiness and revenge

As noted in the previous chapter, few of the assault victims whom we
interviewed were prepared to admit that their own behaviour had contributed to a significant extent to the assault which they had suffered.
Even if they conceded that they had been 'provocative' to some extent –
as in, say, quarrelling with their partner, or giving a 'V' sign to a
motorist who had almost knocked them down – they considered that the
attack which followed was grossly disproportionate to their original
offence. So by and large victims were *not* deterred from reporting by
reason of their feeling responsible for what had happened. Having said
that, some victims had an uncomfortable feeling that their own
behaviour might not bear close scrutiny; they were not necessarily
comfortable about having to explain the sequence of events to the police
(or to a court). For example, Alex Thomas (75) was hesitant about
reporting his assault because he had been drinking heavily and he was

aware that had he not spoken to a youth engaged in a minor act of vandalism he would have been allowed to go on his way unhindered. Gerald Abbott (31), although an ex-policeman, was similarly ambivalent. He had intervened in a quarrel between a youth and a girl – something which he was reluctant to admit even to us but which emerged from the accounts of witnesses. Abbott did admit to a sense that he should not have become involved:

> I shouldn't have been in that position . . . I felt ashamed . . . not ashamed . . . what's the word? (accepts suggestion of 'stigma') . . . of myself for getting involved.

In neither of the above cases did the victim's dissatisfaction with his own role in the incident deter him from reporting. But it might well have done. In the Abbott case, and in that of Sean Bradenham (62), the student 'bouncer' who was assaulted at a university function, the victims were each uncomfortable as what might be regarded as a professional failure -- first in permitting themselves to become involved in a violent incident and second in having been worsted by their opponent. Bradenham was a non-reporter, his desire for vindication failing to overcome his unease at his demonstrated failure to master the bouncer arts.

Non-reporting arising from assault victims' lack of innocence can also be attributed to a generally unfavourable perception of the police – in practice, the two things are closely linked. This is despite survey evidence which has been interpreted to suggest that the decision whether or not to report a given crime is 'incident-specific' rather than rooted in the attitudes of the victim (Sparks *et al*. 1977: 119; Hough and Mayhew 1985: 20). We believe this to be misleading: some people will not report *anything*, no matter how serious (see also Schneider 1976; Shapland *et al*. 1985). It may be that victim surveys are not very successful at identifying people for whom 'dissatisfaction with the police' may be taken to refer not to the police handling of one or two specific incidents but to an anti-police mind-set reflected in the adoption of a way of life which brings that person into regular, hostile contact with the police. For example, George Griffin's most prominent characteristic was his hatred of authority, largely directed against the police. This was despite the fact that the police had been called to his house on numerous occasions and each time had declined the opportunity, generously proffered by Griffin, of charging him with assault. Griffin in fact has no truck with 'the law' in general. He would never go to the police for help (a) because he does not trust them; (b) because he has his reputation to think of; and (c) because he thinks they are useless anyway. His preferred response to this particular assault would be to take the law into his own hands if and when he discovers the identity of his assailants.

Other informants likewise expressed this preference for 'private' justice, claiming that they would take their own reprisals against a known attacker. This was seldom a realistic prospect, it seemed to us. For example, Matthew Howell (49), possessor of a long criminal record, made blood-curdling threats of vengeance against his unidentified attacker, but he was a marginal figure who would have found it hard to locate his assailant and perhaps harder still to turn the tables upon him. We are not ruling out the possibility of revenge attacks, but we suspect that this option is only available to those few assault victims who belong to well-established networks in which such retaliatory violence is sanctioned and encouraged. Even then, as with the 'biker' assaulted by a fellow member of his group, the victim's lowly status in the pecking order may preclude effective action. For the most part, we inferred, victims' threats of vengeance were a reflection of their need to recover from a grievous blow to their autonomy and sense of personal worth. The one exception, in the sense of there being subsequent retaliatory violence, occurred when a male friend of Jane Bond (68), the woman who had been engaged in a drunken brawl with her boyfriend, attempted to seek out the said boyfriend. In the event he fastened upon the man's brother, administering a beating to him instead. So this was a rather poor advertisement for private justice, as it turned out.

Reporting 'domestic' assault

We conclude this chapter with an examination of the factors which may influence the victim of 'domestic' violence when she (as it almost invariably is) has to decide whether or not to call the police. It is difficult to determine whether, in general, violence between intimates is more or less likely to be reported to the police than is 'stranger' violence. One study (Sparks *et al.* 1977: 119) suggested that offences (of all types) committed by friends or family members were rather *more* likely to lead to the police being called, although the authors warned that the decision to report need not indicate a wish that the offender be prosecuted. Other research, both British and American, suggests that victims are *less* likely to report violent conduct on the part of intimates (Gottfredson and Gottfredson 1989: 61; Shapland *et al.* 1985: 48; Mayhew *et al.* 1993: 96). We ourselves encountered high levels of non-reporting in respect of most categories of assault, but it seemed to us that considerations pertaining to 'the relationship' operate, in general, as a barrier both to the involvement of the police in the first place and, thereafter, to the pursuit of criminal prosecution.

The first and most obvious reason for non-reporting is that the victim wishes to preserve a relationship which is still of value to her. Some women were so committed to their violent partner that they could not be persuaded to register a formal 'complaint' even when they had their own independent accommodation and enjoyed the support of their family and the police. Sometimes it was difficult for us to see the value of what appeared a travesty of an intimate relationship, but equally it may have been far from clear what the woman would have gained were she to have reported the incident. The same applied to the one *male* victim of domestic violence whom we encountered. Indeed, he was at pains to check that the police were not routinely informed of those assaults which led to the victim being brought to hospital (as he was). He felt that criminal prosecution would be of no assistance in resolving the under-lying problems between him and his wife. Indeed, he was not concerned with the assault as such and bore his wife no ill-will because of it – he realised that hers was an action taken *in extremis*. All his energies were devoted to seeking a reconciliation.

Along with this preoccupation with the state of the relationship we observed a tendency to play down the violence – even a reluctance to accept that what had happened was really criminal; certainly the victim had no wish for it to be classified in that way. Linda Hutt (34), for example, did not see that this latest assault need upset the pattern of her relationship with her partner which, however unrewarding, still fulfilled some need. The outside observer might view her disinclination to in-volve the police as reflecting her long-term oppression and habituation to her partner's violent conduct, but from Hutt's point of view criminal-isation would have had neither moral nor practical value. As far as she was concerned her troubles belonged in the private realm. The same view was held by other, rather more robust characters. The processes of the criminal law were, as Jane Bond put it, 'too heavy' for an incident which she was prepared to classify as 'just one of those things . . . it was just circumstances . . . we both lost our rag at the same time'. For some women, criminalisation imposed upon an already complex and painful relationship is both burdensome and irrelevant. *We* may think they are oppressed, so that theirs is not a free choice, but we must also consider what benefit they would derive from the criminal process. For the most part, as we shall describe, they would not derive any.

At the same time we must recognise that even where the woman quite clearly *wants* to go to the police, she may not feel able to do so. For anyone trapped in a continuing relationship with their assailant (and this does not only apply in the 'domestic' situation, although that is of course a prime example) the fact of continuing contact may make it impossible to seek help, let alone to sustain a commitment to criminal prosecution. Police protection is inevitably inadequate in providing anything other than the most tenuous sense of security. One example may suffice: Jessie Roberts (37), a professional shoplifter, had suffered repeated beatings at the hands of her boyfriend, causing bruising all over her body. She finally called the police at 3 a.m. one morning. Her boyfriend opened the door and the officers asked to see Roberts. She appeared at a first-floor window, with her boyfriend standing behind her. She felt unable to say anything. Even had she asked for her boyfriend to be arrested, it was inconceivable that Roberts would have sustained her 'complaint'; the physical threat was ever-present. Also, Roberts could not have withstood the moral pressure from her boyfriend, a trainee social worker whose future career would have been damaged by the allegations. It was remarkable that she had found the courage to telephone the police in the first place – that in itself was a reflection of her growing alienation. For women who see no prospect of emotional or physical separation from their violent partner, the call to the police, if made at all, will reflect this need for immediate rescue; but it is unlikely to be the first step on the road to a criminal prosecution.

Another reason why 'domestic' assault does not lend itself to criminal prosecution is that there is likely to have been a history of assault, with the latest incident not necessarily being the most serious. All the women victims of domestic violence whom we interviewed, both reporters and non-reporters, had been attacked by their partner not once but several times. They sought a response which would reflect this history of ill-treatment, rather than a snapshot judgement upon a single (doubtless, according to the assailant, wholly uncharacteristic) violent episode. Amanda Britton (53) was typical in the sense that she did not go to the police when her boyfriend first attacked her and broke her nose; instead she waited until some weeks later, when he threatened to kill her. So she was responding to his generally violent, threatening behaviour. As she said:

> I just got to the stage where I thought somebody else should know about this . . . somebody else should be involved.

In Amanda's case her decision to go to the police was a reaction to her sense of *long-term* injury – not something, in other words, to which the criminal law can readily respond. Likewise Sally Chapman, assaulted by her mother's boyfriend, told us that her motive in going to the police was to punish this man for 20 years of violent conduct, not just for that particular incident (which was comparatively trivial). This desire for some kind of emotional catharsis is unlikely to achieve fulfilment through the processes of the criminal law. The law cannot respond to a history of fear. Nor can it provide a remedy for women who feel they need to act on behalf of other family members as well as themselves. The criminal law can only respond to discrete incidents and that, unfortunately, is only part of the story of domestic violence. Many women, realising this, prefer not to involve the police. Some may be driven to seek their assistance in an immediate crisis, as in the case of Jane Bond who ran shoe-less from the house to make a 999 call, but all too often the pattern of the violence and the motivation for reporting do not meet the prosecuting authority's need for unequivocal evidence in respect of a specific incident.

This may not matter very much if, in going to the police, the woman brings a stop to the violence and achieves a measure of security for the future (Law Commission 1992: 6). As the Law Commission points out, many victims of domestic violence are not primarily concerned with punishment. They may want public condemnation of their assailant and vindication for themselves, in which case they need a criminal prosecution, but even that is not a priority for everyone. Perhaps they simply want removal of the immediate threat. But a simple aspiration (safety) does not necessarily invite a clear-cut course of action, or one that is easily articulated. As Amanda Britton put it:

> People go to the police because they feel safe if they do. That's the whole point . . . it's law and order, isn't it?

Jessie Roberts might say the same, although the police response in her case was almost a parody of ineffectualness. It is possible, nonetheless, that some deterrent effect was achieved. This, certainly, was the reason Roberts called the police; their response should not be judged in terms of its failure to generate a criminal charge since Roberts would not have wanted that in any event.

It is our impression that what many domestic assault victims are seeking is a clear statement that the man's behaviour is unacceptable and wrong. At the same time they may not want him stigmatised by a criminal conviction. This of course sets up an immediate conflict. The responsibility for resolving this conflict is placed at the victim's own door. To give one example, Amanda Britton was asked by the police officer, before he went to arrest her boyfriend, whether she was sure she wished to go through with her 'complaint'. His insistence that she take responsibility for the arrest decision was oppressive to Britton. She felt that she was being asked to commit herself to a course of action which had unknown consequences. Having reported the assault, she felt unequal to doing anything further to 'own' the action. As she put it to us:

It should be the police that press charges as opposed to me.

We suspect in fact that the police may emphasise the victim's responsibility for this decision quite deliberately, as a means of testing her resolve. The Britton case was a good example of the unease experienced by victims who are expected to take responsibility for a prosecution which will subsequently be taken right out of their hands and in which their interests may be considered only as an abstraction.

It is hardly surprising, therefore, that many domestic assault victims, having received some measure of assistance from the police, then decline the prosecutorial assault course which they see ahead. They may do this even where it appears that they will be given every possible support. For example, Linda Hutt had her own council flat; her daughter was almost adult and was in any case in the care of her parents; Hutt had the support of her family and the police in pursuing her 'complaint'; and yet she still withdrew. Samantha Rice (72) likewise had the encouragement of the police; her mother was a co-complainant; she had the support of her ex-husband; her house was her own; but she too declined to support the prosecution of a man who had already been convicted of violence against her.

We shall argue that the reluctance of many women to become involved in a criminal prosecution, or to sustain commitment to that process, is well founded. If the assailant is charged with a criminal offence he will usually be released on bail. Even if such bail is conditional, this cannot guarantee the woman's safety. Furthermore the penalty finally imposed is likely to be modest, and almost certainly non-custodial. In short, the consequences for the assailant bear no relation to the future needs of the victim. This much was understood by those women who had experienced the processes of criminal prosecution in respect of previous assaults. Helen Evans (22) had been forced to leave her home town when her assailant was sentenced to only four months' imprisonment, she having been led to believe that he would receive a much longer term. That experience contributed to her decision not to report her current boyfriend to the police. Other women reported having seen their assailant fined or bound over, which in their view had been ineffective in deterring further violence and might even have exacerbated the situation. Any suggestion that it is desirable for women generally to enlist the criminal law against male violence carried little resonance with these 'experienced' victims.

To conclude, in most of the assaults which we monitored, the act of reporting to the police carried some cost to the victim. In over 50 per cent of cases victim and attacker were involved in a family or sexual relationship, or else they inhabited the same social milieu. Contrast this situation with, say, an assault by one motorist upon another following a car accident. In the latter circumstance there is likely to be no prior personal relationship, in which case the victim's course of action can appear straightforward, the burden upon him comparatively light. There is no requirement for the victim to 'own' the prosecution process; he simply reports the incident to the police, makes a statement, and turns up at court if and when required. The appropriate parallel is *not* with 'domestic' assault but with an offence such as burglary, or with any other criminal offence perpetrated by a stranger. The court appearance may be burdensome, no doubt, but there is no real threat to the victim. But a far more typical *assault* is that in which a decision to report the incident with a view to initiating criminal proceedings carries with it all the baggage of a disrupted relationship, loss of face, risk of exposing the private realm to the public gaze, and the prospect of emotional blackmail and, perhaps, physical intimidation. That, we found, was true of most cases in which there was a reasonable prospect of detection.

Chapter 4

The victim and the police

The police have an acknowledged role as gate-keepers to the justice system. Individual officers confronted with the actuality, the immediate aftermath or the report of violence must exercise their discretion in deciding whether or not to make an arrest (Bottomley and Coleman, 1976; McCabe and Sutcliffe, 1978: 85; Kemp *et al*. 1992: 108–117; McConville *et al*. 1991: *passim*). If they *do* arrest, they have to decide whether or not this is a case for prosecution, for diversion, or for taking no further action. The immediate response is likely to involve not only the comparatively simple consideration 'Has an offence been committed?' but will take into account a number of other factors, each of which may persuade an officer that even though an offence undoubtedly *has* been committed no arrest should follow. It has been asserted that the police, in exercising this discretion, are the most powerful definers of what does or does not become formally recognised as a criminal event (Kemp *et al*. 1992: 17; McConville *et al*. 1991: 141). Views differ as to the legitimacy of this police function (Hough and Mayhew 1985: 3; Gottfredson and Gottfredson 1989: 47–74) and its extent (McConville *et al*. 1991: 90). McConville *et al*. argue that police discretion tends towards the construction of guilt because 'policing culture creates a presumption in favour of prosecution'. Our research, which was victim-based and focused exclusively upon violent crime, led us to a rather different conclusion. We became aware of a strong presumption *against* prosecution, a presumption based on police perception of the difficulties inherent in achieving conviction for crimes of violence. Police awareness of these difficulties leads them to attach considerable importance to the assault victim's commitment to the prosecution enterprise. To a great extent, therefore, the police follow the victim. But they also *guide* the victim down whichever path (prosecution or non-prosecution) they consider appropriate. In this chapter we examine the factors which enter into the police decision to criminalise violent behaviour, and in doing so we consider the extent to which the evidential demands of criminal prosecution lead to a strong emphasis, at this early stage, upon the intentions and wishes of the victim. We shall also consider the degree to which victims are *diverted* from assuming full complainant status; and, third, we shall describe how assault victims may be deflected from 'complaining' (or from 'pressing charges' – it means the same thing) without appreciating that they have been so deflected.

Where police discretion is under discussion two contrary pictures tend to emerge. On the one hand there is the view that individual officers operate a very wide discretionary power: their function in translating 'behaviour' into 'crime' allows them to discriminate against certain classes of victim (for example, female victims of domestic violence) and, equally, against certain classes of offender (say, young male African–Caribbeans). On the other hand, officers themselves will say that they have very little room for manoeuvre. One CID officer engaged on a troublesome case of city centre violence expressed his frustration at being compelled to invest time in such a fruitless exercise:

> Personally I think it's a bit of a waste of time, but they've both made complaints against each other and therefore the police have got to do something. Otherwise, next thing I know, the police discipline department will be coming down on me, asking 'Why didn't you do something about it?'

In this case the officer felt bound by the existence of 'complaints' from two alleged victims. Officers commonly pursue cases which they regard as unpromising or uncongenial (as, for instance, where the victim is a known offender, or is thought likely for some other reason to be an unreliable witness). Their preference in these circumstances, assuming the injuries are not too serious, would be that no one make a 'complaint' and no offence be recorded. But some assault victims prove to be determined complainants, in which case the police will generally feel bound to act. The enthusiasm with which they do so will tend to reflect not the seriousness of the injuries sustained but rather the perceived reliability of the victim/witness and the weight of evidence against the alleged assailant. McConville *et al.* assert that 'victim withdrawal is used to justify non-prosecution when that is the result desired by the police, but when they want to prosecute they ignore the views of the victim' (1991: 123). This is a misleading account, at least in respect of the police response to assault. As we shall describe, the police do indeed deflect some victims and cultivate others, but victim ambivalence and withdrawal is a fundamental reality and something which, in the end, the police can do very little about. The police are powerful in their own way, but victims are powerful in theirs.

THE SIGNIFICANCE OF THE 'COMPLAINT'

The victim of violence turns to the police, broadly speaking, for help. When reporting the incident to the police, or answering questions from an officer at her hospital bedside, she may understand herself to be reporting the harm suffered and asking for police assistance in bringing her assailant to book. In police parlance, however, she will not be 'making a complaint'. The police response to violent crime might be characterised as 'no complaint, no investigation'. This is certainly true of everyday, run-of-the-mill assaults causing injuries of the order of a broken nose, black eye, cuts and bruises. Even where the injuries to the victim merit a s. 20 charge, the importance of the victim's 'complaint' is paramount. The case of pub landlord Timothy Cooper (20) offers a striking example. The police were called immediately after an incident in which Cooper's hand was severely cut by a glass wielded by a customer, Camp. When the police arrived Cooper was being put into an ambulance, his right hand bleeding heavily; Camp was still in the pub and he was pointed out to the police as the assailant. But Camp was not arrested until some days after the attack, the police having by that stage satisfied themselves that Cooper wished to 'complain'.

The distinction between reporting a crime and 'making a complaint' (and thereby signifying commitment to the prosecution process) is unlikely to be appreciated by the lay person. But for the police this distinction is of central importance. They will seldom arrest and prepare a case file for the CPS unless they are confident that they have a victim who is prepared to 'complain'. When the police speak of 'making a complaint' they mean that the victim is prepared to commit herself to a signed statement implicating the assailant, and that she is also prepared, if necessary, to give evidence in court. In all but exceptional cases it is only when they have this assurance that the police act (Cretney *et al*. 1994). The gap which the police create between reporting and 'complaining' has a number of consequences. These are functional for some of the actors in these dramas, dysfunctional for others. First, there is the possibility of misunderstanding – victims may simply not appreciate that more is required of them. Second, the distinction is helpful to the police in that it reflects their operational distinction between being a victim and being a victim who will 'stand up'; they are only interested in the latter. Third, it enables the police to weed out unmeritorious or otherwise dubious victims without their necessarily realising that they *are* being weeded out.

Once we appreciate the central importance which the police attribute to the 'complaint', their response to reported violence can be better understood. For example, violence which is reported by a third party is unlikely to generate an enthusiastic police response. This is because there can be no guarantee that *the victim* (the 'aggrieved') will in fact wish to complain. The attack upon Howard Henderson (11) was brought to police attention by Henderson's girlfriend. Henderson himself would not have wished the police to be involved and in the end he refused to co-operate. This assault gave rise to very serious injury, leading the police, exceptionally in our experience, to pursue an investigation in the absence of a complaint. (Henderson was unable to speak for five days following the attack.) The fact that Henderson eventually declined to make a statement incriminating his assailant might be seen as justifying the police stance. At the opposite pole to assaults reported by third parties are assaults upon police officers. These offer every prospect of 'good process' and so are likely to be seized upon. No doubt this is partly because investigating officers are affronted by the assailant's challenge to police authority, but it is also because police officers can be relied upon not to withdraw their complaint; they are after all professionals and this professionalism extends to their understanding of and commitment to the complainant role.

A statement from the victim is an essential element in the prosecution case. It follows that the police would prefer to have a single complainant, offering unambiguous inculpatory evidence against his or her assailant, rather than two complainants offering contradictory evidence against one another. So we find that one way in which an assailant may escape a criminal charge, especially where the injuries inflicted are relatively minor, is to allege that he was assaulted in turn. We observed several cases run into the sand following the levelling of such counter-allegations. This could be a distressing experience for the person who considered herself the 'true' victim. The young man who 'glassed' Sally Chapman (88) in a gay club alleged, when arrested following a chase, that Chapman had struck the first blow. Chapman recalled her interview with the investigating officer as follows:

> They said 'It's up to you Sally, but he says that you had a go at him first, and you were drunk as well, weren't you?' And I said 'Yes, I was, but I do remember what happened.'

'It's up to you' (whether remembered accurately or not in this instance) is typical police language addressed to a complainant whom the officer considers potentially unsatisfactory for one reason or another and whom he would wish to let the matter drop. Sally Chapman grasped the underlying message and her complaint was accordingly withdrawn.

The centrality of the complaint to the criminal prosecution of assault has been defended on the basis that it confers protection upon victims (Yarsuvat 1989: 241).[1] It nonetheless runs counter to the prevailing understanding, enshrined in law and legal practice, that crime is an offence against the sovereign authority and that it is the state, rather than the individual victim, which determines whether an assailant will be prosecuted (Blackstone 1778: IV: 5). In reality, the police ignore personal violence where the victim does not wish his assailant to be prosecuted. There are exceptions of course, but the police have a tendency to regard most violent incidents as the stuff of private quarrels rather than as harm done to the fabric of society. This does not only apply to assaults which take place in a 'domestic' context.

We shall look more closely at police deflection or nurturing of complaints, but before doing so we shall examine other factors which bear on police decision-making at this stage. These include: the workload of particular police stations and of individual officers (McConville *et al.* 1991: 109); pressure for good police performance in terms of arrest and clear-up rates; the nature of the area in which the incident occurs; whether the violence occurred in public or private; and seriousness of injury. It is perhaps not surprising if, when a young man reports an assault and attempted robbery by persons whom he is unable to describe to the desk officer at a busy inner city police station, no crime is recorded. In such a case the 'character' of the person reporting, the officer's workload, the undesirability of logging minor, undetectable offences, and the nature of the area will each play their part in determining the police response.

The suggestion that the police respond differently to different kinds of victim is of course likely to be resisted by the police themselves. For the most part controversy over police case-handling has concerned perceived unfairness in relation to certain types of *suspect* rather than discrimination in response to victims. (An exception to this has been the intense focus upon the police response to women assaulted by their partners in the home.) Nonetheless it would be remarkable were the police response to be determined *absolutely* by seriousness and detectability. Victims with whom we were in contact ranged from a criminal on the run (in hospital under an assumed name) to an elderly survivor of a World War II prison camp; from a lesbian, heavy drinking resident of St Paul's to a middle-class teacher living in one of the 'best' city areas. They represented all points on the continuum from guilt to innocence, from marginality to solid worthiness. We shall argue, nonetheless, that victim 'worth' in terms of character and social status, while significant, is not the overriding consideration for the police.

Victims least likely to receive an enthusiastic response are those members of the 'rubbish' class who make calls on the police which are 'messy, intractable, unworthy of attention, or the complainant's own fault' (Reiner 1985: 95). These victims will commonly have their private behaviour, their squabbles and disputes, exposed in public – including, very often, to the police. When they do so they are less likely than the rest of us to be accorded victim status. John Wheaton (74) was treated as an in-patient after being knocked unconscious and having his arm broken in a street attack. Wheaton, who is alcoholic and frequents an area of the city populated by other addicts, asked to see a police officer while he was in hospital. Although he was interviewed, no crime was recorded. Wheaton, who claimed (not altogether convincingly) to be able to identify his assailant, spoke bitterly of this and other encounters with the police who took no account of him, he believed, because of his damaged status.

Along with 'rubbish' victims we must consider the impact of 'rubbish' areas. It has been found that in certain problem areas the proportion of reported offences not investigated by the police is much higher than in so-called 'respectable' neighbourhoods (Sparks *et al.* 1977: 157). An officer who worked in the St Paul's district of Bristol referred to this differential response as 'policing by consent'. It was defensible, he suggested, in terms of the differing expectations and understandings of the respective populations:

> People's views, moral standards, and understanding of the law in Stoke Gifford, Little Stoke, Patchway and Hartcliffe are all different. That is why I think we police by consent. We are mindful of community needs.

This puts a respectable gloss upon a policy which few officers would openly defend, as an offence which is decisively criminal in one area becomes only marginally so in another.

We ourselves did not find that the police response to assault was dramatically different by area, but there were certainly instances where assault victims considered that their case had not been pursued because of unfavourable police judgements about *them*. For the most part they lived in the poorer areas of the city, but they also cited other reasons why, in their view, the police had been disinclined to pursue an investigation. Sally Chapman believed she had been discriminated against on several counts:

> I think because it happened in a club they weren't taking it seriously. And as I was drinking as well . . . I thought 'I bet they think I'm a right trouble maker, typical sort of gay woman'. You know, that sort of 'hard woman' image.

The police subsequently declined to charge Chapman's alleged assailant. The reasons given included the assailant's counter-allegations (which were strenuously denied by Chapman) and the fact that Chapman was only slightly injured.

It is not surprising that the operation of police discretion is most evident in relation to 'minor' violence (Chatterton 1983: 220), or that it is in these instances that the perceived character of the victim appears to have most impact. Josephine Macdonald (51) described with some amusement the problem of judgement which she felt she had posed to desk officers at the police station serving St Paul's:

> They were helpful to parts of me. They were helpful to the sort of articulate bit carrying a city council identity card. They were a bit . . . [pause for thought] perhaps the fact that I lived by myself and I didn't have my office suit on, I had sort of punkier clothes on and they were a bit . . . I felt that had I been, well, anything worse – homeless, unemployed – they could have been a lot less sympathetic. But as it was they *were* quite sympathetic in the end, although I did feel that I sort of insisted on it really.

Macdonald, a city council clerk whose dress, hairstyle and perhaps manner hint at her former 'punk' lifestyle, was not easily pigeon-holed. Furthermore she had been assaulted by a former boyfriend, which meant that she was at risk of falling within the 'domestic' classification.

Walter Drobny (32) on the other hand was one of Nils Christie's 'ideal' victims (Christie 1986). Drobny, in his late seventies, had been 'mugged' outside his house by a group of youths, the robbery taking place in broad daylight in a 'respectable' area of the city. He lost a substantial sum of money and he was also seriously, indeed tragically, affected in that his confidence was almost wholly destroyed. There was little hope of detection but the police nonetheless devoted much time and effort to the investigation, conducting house to house enquiries in the area. They also gave time to the personal care of Mr Drobny. The fact that the victim was so badly affected no doubt provides part of the explanation for the determined police response, but so too does the fact that Mr Drobny was archetypally innocent. An exemplary victim attracted an exemplary police response.

Our quantifiable data confirms that there is a relationship between victim status and police and prosecution decisions. This can be seen from Table 4.1.

The likelihood of the assault not being logged by the police, or of the victim not registering a formal 'complaint', or of a complaint being registered but then withdrawn, increases significantly as one descends the social scale. This leaves a higher proportion of middle-class victims whose cases are actually pursued by the police, which explains why more of this group are recorded as failures of detection: a far higher proportion of working-class and (especially) 'rubbish' victims have been weeded out before getting to that point. Nonetheless, these patterns of police/victim interaction at the point of registering a formal complaint feed through to conviction. Of 'middle-class' victims, 32 per cent saw their assailant convicted, as against 25 per cent of victims whom we categorised as 'working class' and 10 per cent of victims in the 'rubbish' category.

Another way of classifying victims is by whether or not they themselves have a criminal record of some sort. Twenty-four (26 per cent) of

Table 4.1 Case progress by victim category

	Middle class	Working class	'Rubbish'
No contact with police	6(21%)	10(23%)	3(15%)
No police record, although the victim claims contact	–	2(5%)	2(10%)
No formal 'complaint', or complaint withdrawn	4(14%)	13(30%)	9(45%)
Complaint sustained, but not detected	8(29%)	5(11%)	3(15%)
Dropped by CPS	1(4%)	2(5%)	1(5%)
Acquitted	–	1(2%)	–
Convicted	9(32%)	11(25%)	2(10%)
Total	28	44	20

the victims in our sample had at least one criminal conviction. Although assaults upon this group were as likely to come to police attention as were assaults upon victims with no record, there was far less likelihood of the police registering a formal 'complaint' – or, if a complaint were recorded, far greater likelihood of its being withdrawn. The figures are given in Table 4.2.

Cases involving 'criminalised' victims achieved a conviction rate of 4 per cent (one case out of twenty-four), whereas there was a 33 per cent conviction rate in respect of assaults upon 'non-criminalised' victims.

These are significant differences, but one cannot immediately say how much the differences are attributable to discrimination on the part of the police and how much to individual case characteristics or to the ambivalence of certain categories of assault victim. It is evident, for example, that the circumstances of some assaults upon damaged victims are such that prosecution is, objectively speaking, more difficult. It is also the case that such victims find it harder to commit themselves to the prosecution enterprise. Nonetheless we accept that initial police assessment of victim worth is a factor, even if the police could argue, with justification, that they are only anticipating these vulnerable cases' future career.

The issue of contrasting police treatment of different categories of victim is most commonly raised in relation to 'domestic' assault.[2] Police officers never fail to register a sense of the peculiar difficulties presented by this type of case:

Table 4.2 Case progress by victim's criminal record

	Criminal record	No criminal record
No contact with police	5(21%)	12(20%)
No police record, although the victim claims contact	1(4%)	3(5%)
No formal 'complaint', or complaint withdrawn	12(50%)	10(16%)
Complaint sustained not detected	4(17%)	12(20%)
Dropped by CPS	–	4(7%)
Acquitted	1(4%)	–
Convicted	1(4%)	20(33%)
Total	24	61

Crime's crime, that's good old black and white, you know what's wrong in that. But domestics, ooh . . .

At the heart of police distaste for 'domestic' calls[3] is the issue of 'the complaint', and specifically the belief that women who report violence are likely subsequently to withdraw their co-operation with the prosecuting authorities. The police understand – or believe they understand – that the relationship between victim and assailant is often such that the woman will not wish, once the immediate crisis has been tackled, to see her partner prosecuted. From the perspective of the police there are also other negative features, including the experience of having to respond repeatedly to calls from the same home with apparently little positive result; the sense that the law is a blunt instrument when brought to bear on domestic circumstances; the perception that even where a conviction is achieved the penalty is likely to be inadequate; the difficulty (and sometimes danger) of intervening in a 'private' situation; the awkwardness, especially for young officers, of dealing with emotional situations beyond their own personal experience; and, possibly, the unpleasantness of removing a man from his home in the presence of young children. Even when we were talking to officers about cases far removed from the domestic sphere, the problematic nature of 'domestics' was frequently mentioned and a contrast drawn between these private, messy, repetitive calls and 'proper' policing.

What is clear is that many women turn to the police *in extremis*, in the hope of immediate relief from violence; they may not have considered the implications of a criminal prosecution. If prosecution follows, even though the woman has given her consent – made her 'complaint' – she may decide to withdraw at a later date. This colours police officers' response to domestic assault, especially if they measure their success in terms of convictions secured – as of course they are encouraged to do within the prevailing political climate. There is also the macho police culture to contend with: the 'social work' aspect of dealing with domestic violence does not come naturally to the majority of officers. It is not what drew them to the job and they are not at ease intruding into a heated emotional atmosphere; their gut instinct is to keep out, even if intellectually they accept that violence in the home is not solely a private matter (Faragher, 1985: 120; Walmsley 1986: 29). Having said this, not all officers are unhappy with this side of policing: some are content to offer immediate practical assistance, recognising that this may be what the woman needs.

Whatever the problems presented to the police by domestic violence, detection is not one of them. Fourteen of the nineteen victims of domestic violence whom we interviewed (73 per cent) gave the police the name and whereabouts of their assailant. This compares with a 32 per cent identification rate in respect of other assaults. Despite the high rate of identification, only 37 per cent of 'domestic' assailants were charged, as against 32 per cent of assailants in other cases. So although a man who attacks his wife or girlfriend is more easily identified than any other category of assailant, he has no greater likelihood of being charged. In 41 per cent of assaults on male victims the assailant was spoken to by the police, whereas in 68 per cent of assaults upon female victims the assailant was spoken to. However, when it came to *charging* the pattern changed. Twenty-three of those who had assaulted male victims (32 per cent) were charged as compared with eight of those who had assaulted female victims (36 per cent). So the 'advantage' enjoyed by female victims in their being able to identify their assailant persisted to the point of having him spoken to, but it then disappeared. The reason for this, according to received police wisdom, lies in the attitude of the complainant. Although women may turn to the police for help in dealing with a violent partner, they will not sustain a commitment to prosecution. The sympathetic police view allows that this may be because of difficulties inherent in the woman's situation, or because the criminal law may not meet her needs;[4] the unsympathetic, probably unspoken but still, arguably, widespread view attributes this vacillation, with its resultant 'waste of police time', to the unsatisfactory nature of women – specifically, those women who have a taste for living with violent men.

So long as successful policing is seen in terms of achieving conviction or, alternatively, of maintaining public order, policing 'domestics' offers only limited satisfaction. There is in effect a mismatch between the needs and expectations of those women who report domestic assault and the working assumptions of police officers who respond to their calls for help. That is not to say that officers do not encourage some women to 'complain'. They do, but they will say that it generally does not get them very far. Louise Purnell (5), the victim of a particularly unpleasant and humiliating attack, was given every encouragement by the police, including the offer (engineered by them) of alternative housing, which she declined. In the end Purnell let it be known that she wanted no further involvement with the police: the assault charges against her boyfriend were dropped when she refused to give evidence at the old-style committal. The exact reasons for her withdrawal from the prosecution process can only be guessed at. They might have included the wish to rebuild the relationship with her boyfriend, or pressure from him. The police officers in this case felt frustrated, but perhaps they had no need to be. Of the victims of domestic violence whom we interviewed, only one expressed herself dissatisfied with police handling of the matter. Jane Bond (68) was one satisfied customer. The police gave her a lift to hospital, ensured that she would be able to go to her parents' house for the night, and offered to go round to her boyfriend's flat, an offer Bond declined. Bond was perfectly content:

> The police were really quite understanding. They said, 'Oh, it'll probably be all right, you'll patch it up.'

So while there are instances where women who wish to instigate criminal proceedings are deflected from doing so by police officers who anticipate that they will retract later on, not all cases of non-prosecution should be regarded as selling the victim short. An officer who, say, advises a victim to consider seeking a civil injunction may have good reasons for doing so, reasons which are not a 'cop-out'. The fact is that the criminal court generally does not deal effectively with domestic violence. Many women, as we shall describe, are profoundly dissatisfied with their experience of criminal prosecution even where a conviction is achieved. The fact that the prosecution must address discrete incidents in what may be a long history of violence is inevitably frustrating for the victim. As far as the police are concerned, they must manufacture out of the complex circumstances of a violent relationship an 'object for policing' (Sheptycki 1992; Kemp *et al.* 1992). This involves removing the incident from its context and this in turn means that the story of the relationship which gave rise to the violence all but disappears. Decisions taken by the police and the CPS, as well as any sentence imposed, are almost bound not to reflect the circumstances of that relationship. The relationship becomes 'the case', limited to a specific offence, defined according to the charge. A police officer who is aware of this may have a justifiably jaundiced view of the value of prosecuting domestic assault even if (or perhaps because) he is sensitive to the needs and wishes of the victim.

Having said this, one must understand that police dependence upon a complainant who is not wholly committed to the prosecution and whose interests diverge from those of the prosecuting authorities is not in any sense confined to domestic assault. On the contrary, while the police and the CPS tend to regard 'domestics' as a distinctively problematic category, we were struck by how much these cases have in common with other 'non-stranger' assaults. The extent to which women victims of domestic violence withdraw their complaints is a matter of some dispute

(Faragher 1985: 16; Sanders 1988). On the basis of our own research we have no doubt that the rate of withdrawal is extremely high, but this is for reasons which we should understand. First, victims may not be free agents; and, second, their needs will often not be met through the criminal process. Sanders (1988) suggests that inaccurate police pre-conceptions about women complainants prejudice their response to domestic violence. We are not convinced that the police perception *is* inaccurate, although we found a similar level of 'unreliability' among other victims of non-stranger assault. The fact is that *all* these complainants are unreliable, and most are unreliable for good reason.

This does not justify a cynical or grudging response, but it is difficult for the police not to be cynical because most measures of their effectiveness are geared to arrest, 'clear-up' and conviction. Given that the criminalisation of assault demands a victim who will remain committed to the prosecution effort, questions of victim *worth* and victim *effectiveness* are bound to be confused. It becomes difficult to distinguish between the moral and the practical since judgements of moral worth may be disguised as pragmatic judgements of a person's endurance and reliability. Businessmen with lap-top computers who have the misfortune to be attacked while driving through a red-light district, young men who get beaten up by night-club bouncers, young women 'glassed' while drinking in a gay club – all may be found wanting. In each case there may be legitimate concerns about the quality of the evidence, but the victim (or the independent observer) will perhaps suspect that the lack of police enthusiasm has something to do with officers' attitudes to gays, to drunken youths, or to those who pay for sex.

Steven Godden (51) was a 'spoiled' victim in that the police strongly suspected he was in St Paul's to pick up a prostitute. He spent a lot of his time in police interview trying to defend himself against suspicion that he had been in the area for that purpose. (His story was that he had taken a wrong turning.) Godden's reason for being in the area was not necessarily material to the fact that he had been robbed, but the police would contend that someone who is not forthright with them is likely to prove a less than satisfactory witness in court.[5] They may anticipate that he will not survive the rough ride of cross-examination, or that he will withdraw before the case gets that far. In this case police fears proved well-founded: Godden failed to turn up for an identity parade (admittedly he had presented himself on two previous occasions, each aborted when the police failed to convene a line-up).

Drunken victims are also likely to be viewed with scepticism. Thirty-one of the assault victims whose cases we followed admitted to having been very drunk at the time they were attacked. Four of these (13 per cent) saw their assailant convicted. By contrast, 25 per cent of cases involving 'moderately intoxicated' victims led to a conviction, as did 35 per cent of cases which involved a strictly sober victim. It is probable that these figures reflect, not a dismissive attitude by police officers towards drinkers, but the fact that where an assault victim is very much affected by alcohol one crucial plank of prosecution evidence cannot be relied upon.

Because the police are interested primarily in cases which can be proved in court, they attach great importance to the victim's own account. Any assault victim will need to convince a police officer that his or her version of the incident is substantially true. It is part of the police officer's job, as he sees it, to exercise a proper scepticism in response to accounts of violence. Officers referred us to cases in which the evidence of independent witnesses had undermined the victim's story, or perhaps had raised question marks against the victim's own behaviour. The most extreme example of police refusal to accept the victim's account was the case of John Enwright (39). As far as the police were concerned Enwright was not a victim but a *suspect*. He had been struck over the head with a breeze-block in the course of a robbery at the depot where he worked: the investigating officers suspected that Enwright was the robber and that he himself had wielded the breeze-block. He was arrested as he left hospital and subjected to a long interrogation. He stuck to his account and the police did not pursue any other avenues. Enwright was not informed of the abandonment of the investigation, as befits his status in police eyes as suspect rather than as victim. This was an extreme case, but not untypical in the sense that the circumstances surrounding an assault are often difficult to penetrate. As a result, imputations of blame, responsibility, and innocence may well be controversial.

Leaving aside the possibility of frank disbelief, there are a number of things which the police might do when presented with a report of an assault which they do not believe is ever going to convince a court. The first is to make no record at all. Of the seventy-three cases in our sample which, according to the victim, were made known to the police, six (8 per cent) were not recorded by them even though the victim gained the impression the assault was being investigated. The fact that minor (and perhaps not so minor) crimes are sometimes 'cuffed' is no secret (Bottomley and Coleman 1976; Chatterton 1983: 203; Sparks *et al.* 1977: 157; Mayhew *et al.* 1993: 16). Victims who live on the margins – the drug user, the alcoholic, the person of no fixed abode – must struggle to overcome a lack of credibility as far as the police are concerned. The victim may feel that he or she has a legitimate grievance; the desk officer on the other hand observes an inarticulate person, possibly of doubtful truthfulness, who is unlikely to be able to provide a coherent or convincing account of what has taken place. If the report is made in a busy station in a locality where low-level violence is commonplace, the temptation not to record an assault may be great. Reiner (1983) has suggested that rules are most likely to be flouted in relation to 'the lesser offender, intellectually and emotionally impoverished'. The same applies, we would suggest, to the lesser victim. But again we should emphasise that 'cuffing' is not simply a response to victim status: seriousness of injury, clarity and plausibility of story, detectability, and the victim's commitment to the prosecution enterprise all play their part.

A second possible response to the 'problem' victim is to discourage him or her from crossing the line from reporting to 'making a complaint'. We noted four cases which were not recorded after the victim herself indicated that she did not want the matter taken further. Describing their role at this point, officers typically speak of 'putting the options'. It is common for people reporting assaults to be told that the decision whether or not to initiate criminal proceedings rests with them. But of course the officer is, in reality, in an extremely powerful position. To an assault victim who may be in a state of some distress, with no knowledge of the criminalisation process and (in cases of domestic violence) equally ignorant of possible civil remedy, the police officer is the expert. The manner in which the officer presents the various options to the victim is likely to determine the choice actually made (Faragher 1985: 117). For example, in explaining the courses open to a woman reporting domestic assault the officer may make plain the difficulties inherent in criminal prosecution, the *burden* upon the woman, and her responsibility to the prosecuting authorities. Undue emphasis upon this burden, without corresponding encouragement to the woman to pursue her complaint, could be construed as a failure to offer support where it is most needed. The police, on the other hand, see it as justified realism.

This also applies to assaults in other contexts. Take, for example, the case of Brian Miller and his brother-in-law (38) who were attacked and concussed by unseen assailants late one night. The officer who interviewed Miller the following day told him that it was up to him whether or not he wished to 'complain', but that there was very little point in continuing with the case. Miller agreed to 'drop the charges' (as he put it) and in so doing enabled the officer not to record the offence. In this instance the options were indeed presented, but in such a way as to allow the officer to 'cuff' a most unpromising case. If Miller's injuries had been severe, both victim and officer might have had fewer 'options' available.

Another possible strategy is to require the victim to do the work – that is to say, to gather further evidence to support an assault charge. Robert James (63), a student who was bruised and cut in a street attack witnessed by his friends, was asked to gather his witnesses and take them to a police station at some distance from his home in order that they might all make statements. As it happened James possessed a car and he proved willing and able to comply with the police request. This kind of delegation of responsibility from the investigating officer to the victim is principally employed, we believe, to test the victim's commitment to the process. It is superficially reasonable, at least in the case of a comparatively affluent young man who has the means to ferry his friends about, but in practice it is likely to sound the death knell of the case. Kevin Pilcher (27) was interviewed in hospital where he was recovering from a broken jaw. He was asked to attend Central Bristol police station on his discharge from hospital and to bring with him the various friends and acquaintances from the southern fringe of the city who had witnessed the attack upon him by pub bouncers. Pilcher was willing to make a statement, or so he claimed to us, but he was unable to persuade his witnesses – some of whom he did not know well – to make the five-mile journey to the city centre. Given that Pilcher himself had served a sentence of imprisonment for assault, and that the witnesses all lived on an estate notoriously hostile to the police, it was a little fanciful to imagine that Pilcher would ever succeed in this proposed rounding up. In fact, because he could not persuade his witnesses to attend, he himself did not bother to make a formal statement. There was thus no investigation in this case (although Pilcher had given the name and workplace of the 'bouncer' to the police) because the officer was awaiting a formal complaint from the victim and concluded that he was not interested in making one:

> We've got other things to do, and if the person doesn't co-operate . . . doesn't come in when he says he's going to, you think . . . well does he really want to go anywhere with this. And after making several phone calls . . . [he tails off].

When asked why he had not pursued the witnesses himself, the officer replied:

> Initially we had to get a statement of complaint from [Pilcher], because there's no point in pursuing the matter unless we get a statement from the aggrieved.

So the failure to get a 'complaint' from Pilcher when he was lying in hospital with his jaw wired, allied to the requirement (as Pilcher understood it) that he produce his own witnesses, led to this investigation being aborted. The officer concluded that this was because Pilcher . . .

> never came up with the goods. It's his decision at the end of the day to call it off . . . it was never mine. I was quite prepared to go ahead and deal with it.

This is true up to a point, but it was never Pilcher's decision to 'call off' the investigation, and the officer was only prepared to 'deal with it' if Pilcher were to perform the somewhat unlikely feat of corralling his own witnesses.

Finally there is the possibility, even following the victim's registering of a formal 'complaint', of further testing the victim's commitment through delay. Especially in cases of 'domestic' assault the investigating officer may anticipate the woman's withdrawal. Mindful of this, he may be in no hurry to make contact with the alleged assailant. This again may be viewed as a legitimate tactic, enabling the police to 'test' hesitant complainants, but it could equally be seen as imposing an inappropriate burden upon a vulnerable person. Amanda Britton (53) had wanted her ex-boyfriend arrested speedily so that he might be 'taken away, stuck in a cell for a night and made to realise what he's done'. She gave the police both his home address and his place of work. When the boyfriend, Morris, had still not been arrested four weeks after the assault was reported, Britton tried to discover what was going on. She was told that there had been a delay because the arrest would have to be handled from a neighbouring police station covering the area in which Morris lived. She was also asked whether she was 'really sure' that she wanted Morris arrested. Britton said she *was* sure, although she told us shortly after this that she was beginning to have doubts. Five weeks after the assault Morris was arrested. However, he made counter-allegations against Britton and this led to his not being charged; instead both he and Britton were summonsed. This prompted the couple to contact one another, whereupon they agreed to drop their respective allegations. The WPC who handled the conclusion of the case remarked that:

> It probably happened for the best really. Just another case of heat of the moment.

This took no account of the fact that Britton had a legitimate complaint against Morris, who had broken her nose. Perhaps Morris should have had to suffer what Britton wanted him to suffer – a night in the cells. But time was allowed to pass and matters resolved themselves without any recognition of the fact that Britton had been the victim of an assault. She herself felt that she had been tested by the police in a way which her obvious status as a victim did not warrant. The delay in arresting Morris and the police emphasis upon the importance of her role as complainant led to a weakening in her resolve. So what appears to have been a dilatory and sceptical police response induced the lack of commitment to the prosecution process with which officers sometimes stereotype women complainants.

If the above are some of the ways in which victims may be discouraged from pursuing their complaint, there are also circumstances in which the police appear anxious – one might even say desperate – to ensure that a complaint is forthcoming. This might be a reflection of the gravity of the assault, but pressure on the victim to complain also arises where the usual order of events – complaint, followed by arrest – is reversed, so that the police find themselves in the awkward position of having made an arrest before the victim confirms that he or she is prepared to co-operate – in other words, an arrest, but no case. This commonly arises where the police have arrested someone in response to a perceived threat to public order. Complex and volatile public order situations pose considerable problems for the police and we noted three apparently contradictory responses. The first of these, as we have indicated, is a search for complainants in the wake of arrests; the second is the 'disappearance' of victims in light of the police preoccupation with restoring order; and the third is the deployment of assault charges with minimal prospect of conviction in the hope of using them as part of the currency of a plea-bargain.

We observed a few cases in which arrest generated its own momentum, with, for example, the police visiting victims in their homes in the hope of persuading them to make statements, the supposed assailant having already been arrested by officers called to the scene of a public disturbance. Some of these 'victims' had suffered but modest injury and would have been quite prepared to let the matter lie. For example, when police arrested Philip Cleese (71) late one night following a violent incident outside the Bristol Royal Infirmary, they attempted to persuade his two alleged victims to repair to Bristol Central police station after they were discharged from the A & E Department in order that they might make statements. They declined to do this (it was 2 a.m.), but other officers visited them at home the following day and statements were duly taken. So we observe that once a person has been arrested the prosecution momentum which is thereby generated creates a pressure on the police to locate someone who is prepared to 'complain'.

In other public disturbances the police may be so preoccupied with restoring order and containing damage (McConville *et al.* 1991: 31) that assaults may be lost sight of. It may be that the disturbance is contained and the police are content to make no arrests; or else they may consider *only* the public order dimension and arrest and charge on that basis (Sanders 1988). The identification of assault victims, and of assailants, may be low on their list of priorities. Matthew Collins (35) was one young man who felt he had suffered as a result of this. The police had been called by a publican following an encounter between Collins and a former secondary school class-mate, Steven Patten, outside a pub. A physical confrontation in the street had led to both young men crashing through a shop window. Now they were sitting inside the pub, surrounded by rival 'supporters'. Collins' account of the incident was that Patten had first yelled abuse at him and then, unprovoked, had rugby tackled him so that both youths had fallen through the window. The police officer (a young probationer) had arrived at the pub to find, as he later explained, two rival groups of young men. His first duty, as he saw it, was to disperse the crowd. Accordingly he asked them to leave the pub. The witnesses to the 'assault', if that is what it was, accordingly disappeared, suggesting that the officer had not contemplated the possibility of an assault charge. In the event Collins and Patten were each charged with criminal damage and bound over to keep the peace, having promised to compensate the shopkeeper for his broken window. An assault charge against Patten was considered, but rejected for lack of evidence. Collins' right hand was badly cut in the incident and a tendon severed, with the result that his future as a plasterer was put in jeopardy. Patten incurred only minor injury. Clearly the circumstances surrounding the 'assault' were murky; a prosecution might not have succeeded. Collins, however, was of the view that he had been the innocent victim of his former school-mate's aggression and yet had found himself in court as a defendant rather than as a victim.

Finally, we observed that assault charges can be deployed as part of a 'belt and braces' approach following a major incident. This happened in the case of Patrick Dashwood and his friends (3). These young men were very badly hurt, and it was known that the damage had been inflicted by a group of bouncers from two neighbouring establishments. But it was not easy for the police to establish which of the bouncers had been prime movers in the assault and which had contributed only marginally. The victims had been knocked unconscious and so could not identify their assailants. Other witnesses had had only a partial or distant view. The police charged three of the defendants with both s. 18 assault and violent disorder. In due course the defendants 'pleaded' to the charge of violent disorder and the s. 18 charges were dropped. It is easier to prove public order charges than it is to prove assault, so it is quite common for assault charges to form part of the currency of the plea bargain. It has been argued (McCabe and Sutcliffe 1978: 86; Sanders 1988) that this allows the law to give better protection to male victims since their victimisation is likely to occur in a public place. This rather begs the question of whether criminalisation does in fact confer protection upon victims, but it is true that the availability of public order charges means that the police have a second string to their bow when responding to violence in these circumstances.

SERIOUSNESS AND THE LIMITS OF POLICE DISCRETION

In responding to assault the police make a pragmatic distinction between those offences which are capable of proof in court and those which are not. This distinction is also made in respect of other offences, such as rape (Blair 1985: 54). Hence the importance of the 'complaint', to which we have paid so much attention in this chapter. If follows that seriousness of physical injury is not, as might be thought, of great significance in determining whether or not the police pursue an investigation. This is at odds with the conclusion reached by other researchers. For example, Gottfredson and Gottfredson (1989: 258) argue, on the basis of research material reviewed in their book, that:

> The power of [seriousness] is . . . difficult to overestimate; it survives to be used again and again, despite continuous truncation and selective samplings of the seriousness distribution. At each stage, the gravest dispositions are reserved for those cases, among those that are passed on from earlier stages, that are judged or classified the most serious.

Chatterton (1983: 216) likewise observes that police discretion is greatest in respect of less serious cases. Both these statements are true up to a point, but they are nonetheless liable to mislead. Grave physical injury *does* influence the police, but apart from the very top and bottom of the seriousness scale the degree of harm inflicted is more or less incidental to the police decision to investigate an incident, to arrest, and to charge.

The point about very serious or well-publicised assaults, viewed from this perspective, is that they bring pressure on the police to behave in uncharacteristic ways. Police officers respond emotionally to serious harm inflicted upon vulnerable people. They are also influenced by the publicity given to a particular offence. While this is most obviously true of those crimes which make national headlines, it can also be true of incidents which attract only local publicity. As one officer commented, referring to an attack upon a man in a car park on a Sunday morning:

> Something had to be done. I mean we would have been seen in a very bad light if it got into the press that somebody'd received a fractured skull at half past ten in a car park on a Sunday morning – we wouldn't have been very popular!

Perceived gravity and publicity *do* therefore influence the police, perhaps inducing them to proceed with an investigation even though they know that their one source of evidence, the victim, cannot be relied upon. This might be viewed as an attempt to adhere to the 'offence against society' model upon which our criminal justice system is supposedly based and to buck the 'complainant' model upon which, we argue, the prosecution of assault is *in reality* based. One might see it as *testing* the offence against society model in a way that it is not normally tested. In fact it tests it to destruction, thereby tending to confirm that the police are justified, practically speaking, in focusing so much of their attention upon 'the aggrieved'. This can be demonstrated with reference to those few cases in which, responding to the seriousness of the injuries inflicted, the police mounted an investigation either without waiting for a complaint or in the absence of a firm commitment from the complainant. Howard Henderson (11) had sustained a multiple fracture of the jaw. A knife was used in the attack which happened, apparently, because Henderson's assailant believed Henderson to be trespassing on his drugs patch. Over the following five days police officers expended considerable time, effort and paperwork on this case. It all came to nothing when Henderson himself refused to 'complain' – that is to say, to make a statement implicating his assailant. The investigating officer summed up the case as:

> . . . a lot of hard work, a lot of paperwork. And to sum it up quite frankly – for bog-all. And it even goes a stage further than that. That is why some of them think it is safe to go on committing offences out there, because there aren't going to be any witnesses. They can get away with the fact that there's a good chance that the aggrieved party won't go to court.

In other cases, such as those of Barker (10), Paxman (6), Freeman (4) and Purnell (5), the police brought pressure to bear on the victim to make a statement despite his or her strong reservations. In none of these cases was there any doubt as to the identity of the assailant. But each prose-cution failed following the victim's withdrawal of co-operation with the prosecuting authorities. Timothy Paxman had made it plain to the officers called to the scene that he wanted no police involvement. Only because of the severity of Paxman's injuries was the case pursued. The officer in the case explained:

> Our feeling was, from the description of the attack, had he not had his arms up to protect his head he would have received those blows about the head and potentially we could have been looking at a murder.

Although the investigating officer was aware of Paxman's vulnerability as a witness (he had been a drug addict since he was 14 and was now living in fear of his assailant) he pressed on with the case. But once in court Paxman declined to identify his attacker and the case collapsed.

Henderson, Barker, Paxman, Freeman and Purnell had all been badly hurt. The police pursued their investigations in determined fashion, despite the obvious problems. In each case the stakes were high, but in each case, also, the victim was vulnerable to intimidation from the assailant and/or pressure from within his local community. We are talking here about very vulnerable people whom the police can do little to protect. The police did not reject them, but nor did they feel they could offer the victim the kind of support which might conceivably have made a difference to the final outcome.[6] We conclude therefore that while seriousness is central to decisions concerning charge and sentence, victim resolution – which includes police *perception* of victim reso-lution – generally overrides seriousness in determining the progress of the case.

Chapter 5

The police and the demands of the legal process

In this chapter we examine the way police practice in investigating assault is influenced by what officers understand to be the standards of evidence required by the CPS and, thereafter, by the court. It will be seen that we take issue with the image of all-embracing police power presented by McConville *et al.* (1991: *passim*). At least in relation to the police investigation of assault, the evidential demands of the CPS and the court are internalised by officers, influencing every stage of the process and largely determining which cases are pursued and which are dealt with perfunctorily or not at all.

We have seen that many cases do not proceed beyond the initial report to the police because the victim declines to 'make a complaint'; more commonly it will be a police officer, either uniformed or CID, who decides that a case will not repay further investigation. Sometimes this decision is influenced by the officer's perception of the character or reliability of the complainant, but in making it the officer will believe that he or she is weighing the likelihood of achieving conviction. That is the key test, towards which all other judgements contribute. Having said that, there are some cases which, while they present formidable detection problems, attract considerable police effort. There are certain identifiable features which contribute to making these cases a hard nut which it is nonetheless worth attempting to crack.

Before we examine factors which influence police assessments of detectability, we offer an account of 'good practice' – that is to say, routine, standard practice – as this is perceived by officers themselves. Here is one officer's account of what he believed to be the 'copy-book' response to a reported assault:

> To do the job correctly I'd say that if you've got somebody who can give you a description of the offender and he (the victim) has got

visible injuries, then we're told to make a crime report because it's a crime that's coming to you, a reported crime. . . . And then, if he's reporting an assault, you're looking to see what grade of injury they've got. If it's not visible then we're probably talking about a common assault, which we can deal with, but generally speaking you'd advise them to take their own action. But [in this particular case] I was looking at an ABH with visible injuries, so the least I'd expect to do was to take a statement, arrange for photographs of the injuries, get a doctor's statement, and then get them to look through a photo album. Then we're armed with everything we need, rather than pestering them at a later stage, or later on when their injuries have gone down or there's nothing visible. Then, if we pick somebody up, yes, they've had their injuries photographed, yes, we've got a statement, and there's a crime report. That's basically it. But at the end of the day we're only as good as the information we get. If they can't identify anybody and no witnesses can, that's as far as it's going to go.

This account identifies the main factors in the ideal police response: (i) the need to take reported crime seriously; (ii) the need to identify the nature of the harm done (to categorise it according to legal definitions in order to determine the charge); (iii) the need for evidence, starting with the victim's identifying (or providing a good description of) his assailant; and the need to prepare a case file.

In practice, as one might expect, the police response can be much less efficient than this. The painstaking, well-ordered response to reported assault is the exception rather than the rule. For example, an alleged assailant will commonly be arrested at night by one officer, who might then interview the victim and secure a 'complaint', leaving the assailant to sober up in the cells for some hours. The alleged offender might then be interviewed by a second officer, whose knowledge of the incident may well have been gleaned through oral communication from a *third* officer. This is what happened, according to the arresting officer, in the case of Annie Cresswell (59), possibly accounting for the disappearance of the victim's allegation that she had been threatened with a knife. In fact the knife itself, which had been handed in by the arresting officer, also disappeared. Likewise when Sally Chapman's stepfather, John Dwyer, was arrested (60), the *arresting* officer had not interviewed Chapman. Dwyer then spent the night sobering up before being interviewed by a *third* officer. Any sense of the identity of an incident is likely to be dissipated as the case is passed around in this fashion. Additionally, no one officer will be sufficiently well informed to feel a sense of responsibility towards the victim. In this case a prosecution was brought, but dropped by the CPS on Dwyer's first appearance before the magistrates. Two months later Chapman had heard nothing and was still anxiously awaiting a trial. A second example of a case which suffered by being passed from officer to officer was the potentially lethal attack upon Michael Fleming (7). The detective constable eventually given responsibility for this case admitted that it had not been well managed, passing through five pairs of hands in ten days. The initial failure to record the incident as an assault was compounded by disconnected police case management thereafter. The resulting delays seriously handicapped the investigation when it did eventually get off the ground.

Despite this evidence of confused or inefficient police case management, the officers whom we interviewed (especially CID officers) asserted with some confidence that assaults, in general, were not difficult to detect. The *actual* detection rate among our sample of ninety-three cases is given in Table 5.1.

The figures bear out officers' claims that by the standards of offences such as burglary, assaults are not unduly difficult to detect. This was explained by one experienced CID officer as follows:

> There are times when people will say that we've done sweet f.a., but I can tell you that that is *never* the case with these serious assaults. We detect the majority of them – and most of them with the help of the public. They're *far* easier than burglaries, because most often people are around – they take place in pubs, clubs, in the home, or on the roads . . . I feel quite confident that we're very successful in detecting them . . . it's the car thefts and the burglaries that we're no good at. But serious assault – those are the ones we detect. And I don't think the public should have any fear that we're useless at it . . . we're not . . . we're very good at it.

As this officer acknowledged, the high detection rate in respect of

Table 5.1 The detection rate among our research sample

Police not informed	19(20.4%)
Police informed but offender never identified	23(24.7%)
Offender identified but not contacted	7(7.5%)
Offender spoken to by police but not charged	13(14%)
Offender charged	31(33.3%)
Total	93(100%)

assault depends very largely upon the victim's own ability to identify his or her assailant. Given that so many assaults take place between familiars, or between people moving in the same social milieu, this need not present any great difficulty. As officers acknowledged, the problem generally lay not in identifying the assailant, but in persuading key witnesses (especially the victim) to make statements and, if necessary, to give evidence in court. But detection – if we accept that the police being informed of the identity of the assailant merits the use of that term – can be quite straightforward. The unfortunate paradox is that it is precisely in those cases where the police have least difficulty in identifying the assailant that they tend to have *most* difficulty in bringing the case to court. This was one Detective Sergeant's view:

> I don't think assaults are that difficult to detect. I mean, I don't know what our detection rate is on assaults in this force, or even on this division, but I believe it's relatively high. A high percentage of assaults are committed by people that are known to the victim: domestic, neighbours – and then you get your Saturday night pub fights. And nine times out of ten that is a group of lads from one part of the city, two lads have gone out and had their few pints, can't get into a club, can't find a woman, so they give someone a whacking. And we're very fortunate because we're rather isolated here – they've either got to get a car or a taxi in order to get home, so they get arrested within the area where the assault took place. So most of the time you've either got witnesses or someone who's able to say 'I know who it was'. Whereas you don't have that for street robberies or burglaries. If it's confined to a pub, there's always someone who's got a rough idea who the bloke is, or somebody's come in – 'he's a regular here' – or whatever. But they're harder to get to court, yes.

Of course some assaults – the ones the police like best – are both easy to detect *and* easy to get to court. The ideal conditions for 'good process' in respect of assault charges would appear to be:

- a staunch complainant;
- a readily identifiable assailant;
- the absence of any prior personal relationship, particularly one of intimacy;
- serious, clearly visible injuries; and
- reliable witnesses.

If the assailant is a particularly worthwhile 'catch' from the police point of view, so much the better.

Troublesome assaults are ones which display the contrary features. Experienced detectives told us that there were many cases where they knew from the outset that the chances of successful prosecution were slim. In the words of one:

> You can look at a job, read the statements, and you *know*, from the word go, that you haven't got much of a chance of detecting it at all.

There were two main reasons for such pessimism: first, a lack of evidence such that it was unlikely that the police would be able to identify the assailant or prove a case against that person; and second, problems emanating from the relationship between victim and assailant.

The first of these difficulties is well understood and was reflected in many of the cases which we followed. For example, the police have an almost impossible job in prosecuting late-night city-centre violence – unless they happen to be present in force, which they usually are not. There is also the fact that most potential witnesses will have been drinking and so will be uncertain as to precisely what happened – or at least, it may be impossible to get someone to give an account which appears sufficiently authoritative and clear-headed to secure conviction. The detective investigating the Nigel Jenks assault (30) viewed the enquiry as almost inevitably abortive. The same may be said of street muggings such as were suffered by Howell (49) and Davies (52): there is little prospect of success given the victim's inability to make a positive identification. The best hope of a 'clear-up', as happened in the Howell case, was to put the assault to a convicted robber serving a prison term for other, similar offences.

The second kind of difficulty is less well understood, but it became evident in the course of our case monitoring that the fact that so many assaults involve acquaintances, or intimates, assists in *detection* but undermines *prosecution*. This is recognised as presenting a particular problem in the context of 'domestic' violence, but it is also apparent where victim and assailant have some other kind of social relationship – most notably, one involving a power imbalance such as one may observe between drug user and supplier. It was in relation to the assault on Timothy Paxman (6) in the St Paul's district of Bristol that the investigating officer commented:

> In an area like this you begin to think 'Oh Christ, not another one' – because it's one of those jobs – although there's a complaint on paper you think you're not gonna get a successful prosecution.

In this instance, the officer explained, Paxman's drug addiction was such that he was bound to remain in contact with his assailant or his associates in order to secure his supply. He was not going to be able to stand up in court and give evidence – or if he did, he would be a terrible witness: 'One way or another, we'll have problems when it comes to the prosecution.' The officer's prediction proved to be correct. Once in court Paxton declined to identify his assailant. The officer observed: 'A typical job for this area.'

A related difficulty in this kind of case is the fact that the victim may lack 'innocence' so that, even were he to withstand the rigours of the trial process, his credibility as a witness would be undermined. The officer in the Paxman case had worked in St Paul's for seven years and enjoyed doing so, but in that time, or so he claimed, he could not recall going to court with a case in which there was no difficulty with the complainant or with other witnesses:

> If it's a rape, my victim is usually a prostitute . . . it's always jobs like that, and there's always problems.

In this officer's view, juries were inclined to look sceptically upon assault victims such as Timothy Paxman, thinking:

> You've brought this on yourself, mate . . . if you didn't want that to happen, why were you in St Paul's?

According to the police, many assault victims in St Paul's could be presented, by the defence, as of dubious character for one reason or another. Given that the evidence in the case might boil down to one person's word against another's, it was unhelpful for the victim to be no more 'respectable' than his alleged assailant. This was a feature of the David Freeman case (4). Freeman, although a young man, had a formidable criminal record, comparable to that of two of his assailants and *more* heinous than that of the leader of the gang who had tortured him. He had also told a number of blatant untruths in his original statement to the police. Freeman proved remarkably resilient in standing up to cross-examination, both at the old-style committal and the eventual trial, so the fact that he feared further attack – indeed, that he feared for his life – did not prevent his giving evidence on two occasions. The trial was in fact aborted because it could not be concluded before the judge was due to go on holiday, thereby denying us an opportunity of discovering whether Freeman's evidence, despite his damaged status, would be sufficient to secure conviction. As might have been predicted, Freeman did not put in an appearance at the *second* trial, which meant that the investigating officer's gloomy prognostications proved in the end to be well-founded. This was a case with several negative indicators so it was rather poignant that but for a somewhat exceptional *procedural* buffeting it might have survived them all. Instead, two of the three defendants spent 12 months in custody only for the prosecution, in the end, to offer no evidence against them.

THE DEMANDS OF THE PROSECUTION PROCESS

It is argued by McConville *et al.* (1991: 54) that prosecution is not the sole, or even the main, goal of many arrests. The police may use the processes of arrest, detention and trial as a demonstration of their own power to impose 'law and order' rather than, necessarily, to achieve successful prosecution in the individual case. Thus from the police point of view it may not matter that the defendant is acquitted or that the case never gets to court: if the object is to impose authority and achieve order, that can be achieved through the process of arrest and the accompanying demonstration of police power . . . the process *is* the punishment. This emphasis upon the police service's (and the individual officer's) strategic goals echoes Chatterton's claim that an arrest for assault is not a 'good' arrest from the officer's point of view since it is unlikely to contribute to the clear-up of other offences; the officer who arrests a burglar is playing a more effective role in the local 'fight against crime' than is his colleague who arrests a wife-beater or a drunken youth (Chatterton 1983: 204).

We would not suggest that this view of police motivation and practice is without foundation, but in our view McConville and his colleagues give too much weight to one particular insight while contradictory material is treated dismissively. We ourselves observed cases which attracted more police effort than appeared justified simply on the basis of seriousness or detectability. To give one example, the police devoted considerable time and effort to the apparently hopeless investigation of the assault upon Sandra Hind (36), perpetrated outside one of the city's better known nightclubs for young people. That club was in bad odour with the police, who had attempted to have its licence revoked and who might therefore have welcomed the chance of pinning another act of violence upon the club and its customers. But this kind of incidental organisational objective was not a feature of the police response in the majority of cases which we followed. It was much less striking than officers' awareness of the evidential standards imposed by the CPS and courts. For the most part they geared their efforts to meeting those standards.

McConville *et al.*'s account of the reality of police work presents the police as manipulative and powerful, bending rules and undermining the structures of legality and legitimacy in pursuit of effective prosecution. An alternative view, to which we would subscribe, acknowledges police power to define the suspect population but also gives emphasis to the constraints imposed by a lack of available evidence and by CPS requirements. Victims and witnesses make cases just as much as do the police. The police do indeed seek to build and control the prosecution case, but their power to do so is limited.

Reference has already been made to the relationship between moral and pragmatic judgements as to victim 'worth'. Police officers whom we interviewed stressed the evidential problems which arise where witnesses are reluctant to make statements or cannot be found; where the victim's account is contested; or where the victim is judged unreliable or unlikely to make a good impression in court. Police detection work is not conducted in a vacuum – it is highly contingent upon the rules imposed from above. The police response is often inadequate if viewed in terms of their enthusiasm for righting wrongs. The police do not behave like the knights of old: their response to violent incidents is constrained (certainly in their own eyes) by CPS requirements and court guidelines. This helps to explain why officers can appear unenthusiastic in their conduct of cases which, to a layperson's eyes, seem eminently detectable.

We are aware of suggestions that the police should be subject to greater CPS control because of their excessive zeal for prosecution. At the same time, even without such control, many assault victims experience what they perceive to be an inadequate response from the police. We ourselves observed a lack of police enthusiasm in cases where unequivocal evidence was not easily come by and a considerable time commitment demanded. In many of these cases the victim was persuaded that it was not worthwhile to 'complain'. Equally, our experience of following assaults which went to trial confirmed how difficult it is to achieve a conviction in anything other than the most straightforward case. It is not surprising if there is a lack of police zeal in pursuing investigations where the officer knows that the alleged offender is unlikely to be prosecuted, let alone convicted.

The corollary of this emphasis upon a case's prosecutorial worth is that trivial cases, if detectable, may be rigorously pursued. Patrick Tapnell, who was convicted of threatening behaviour towards Alan Small (90), a university student, was identified by two student friends of Small who had been with him in the pub when a general mêlée broke out. The witnesses were sober (although Small himself was not) and they identified Tapnell after police officers had escorted them on a tour of the area. Tapnell was immediately arrested and, seven months later, convicted. Small had been assaulted, but the police acknowledged that Tapnell was not the assailant. We have to ask: why was he prosecuted? We believe that it was because this case represented 'easy process' for the police. Responding to certain cues, the police response was triggered. No test of gravity was applied, nor was there any measure of relative culpability as between 'victim' and 'offender'. The cues which triggered this Pavlovian response were: public disorder requiring an immediate response; clear identification by two sober witnesses of good character (Small himself could not remember anything); a suspect willing to inculpate himself beyond all reasonable expectations (Tapnell admitted that he had *felt like* 'having a go' at Small); and a victim who, if not much use as a witness, was at least willing to sustain a 'complaint'. The police officers in the case admitted to us that they might well have nudged Small in the direction of not registering this complaint, but they chose not to do so – probably because they had already made an arrest. Presented with what even the police thought was a weak case, the CPS went ahead, with the result that considerable time and money was spent on prosecuting Tapnell for a minimally violent act within a context of general disorder. He was found guilty in the magistrates' court: a shocking outcome for a man who had never previously faced a criminal charge.

In contrast, serious incidents involving behaviour which is far more culpable might attract a hesitant, ambivalent response from the police. The explanation for this lies partly in overt problems of detection, partly in assessments of the victim's character and class, and in part it is a response to the context of the violence. These factors contribute, albeit in an intuitive way, to a police sense that a given case is never going to get anywhere. Accordingly, some very bad assaults attract minimal investigative effort. The 'mugging' of the businessman, Steven Godden, who the police suspected was in St Paul's in search of a prostitute (50), was one example; the attack upon Michael Fleming, also in St Paul's (7), was another. Fleming was able to give us (researchers) the name and address of a witness, but the police had not been able to follow up this 'lead'. The investigating officer explained:

> He's told me one name – a Christian name – but he hasn't been able to identify him such that we know who it is. We *think* we know who it is, but we haven't been able to get hold of that person, and if it is who I think it is, I don't think we would have any luck there. It's not the done thing for them to be seen to collaborate with us . . . he's

certainly not come forward, and there's nothing to say that he did in fact witness anything more than the other people who were there.

It is unlikely that anyone beaten nearly to death with a brick would find this response wholly satisfactory. In Godden's case the police effort, or lack of it, was influenced by the fact that one of the alleged assailants was already on remand in respect of other offences: the police appeared content that the assault on Godden should be 'put to' this prisoner and thus cleared up without the effort (and risk of failure) attached to a separate prosecution.

Other, less serious and less obviously detectable cases drew a painstaking (but fruitless) response from the police. The fact that the principal yardstick of detectability was overridden in these instances can be attributed to secondary offence characteristics of victim character and area. Among this group was the assault upon Walter Drobny (32). This was a distressing incident, but there were no witnesses; the victim was perhaps insufficiently robust to face the ordeal of giving evidence in court, or even of identifying his assailants; and there was little prospect of any evidence turning up. Nonetheless the investigation stayed alive for five weeks. It was evident that as an elderly, blameless victim Drobny attracted considerable police sympathy and this, perhaps allied to the perception that the attack had taken place in a 'respectable' area, contributed to a vigorous response. One might conclude therefore that while detectability is the chief determinant of police effort, it is not *all*-important because the police are influenced by judgements of victim worth which extend beyond the pragmatic assessment of that person's viability as a witness.

The police are also concerned, in an image-conscious age, with their corporate public persona. The detection of certain crimes has a symbolic value for the police. As a result, considerable resources may be devoted to high-profile cases while others, perhaps equally serious, attract minimal police effort. Cases which do not register with the public (although they may be traumatising for the victim) are less likely to attract investigative effort and resources. It is difficult to establish a clear association between offence visibility and police effort because the most visible cases tend also to be the most serious, but our observation of the police response to run-of-the-mill assaults suggests that these rank fairly low on their list of priorities. One explanation for this might be that a failure to detect would do the police little public harm. It has been suggested that where injuries receive public attention by virtue of the victim seeking hospital treatment, the police response will be influenced by the greater risk of public criticism in those cases (Chatterton 1983: 218). Having studied a group of cases in which the victim had in every case sought hospital treatment we are less convinced that the police view hospital referral as contributing in any significant degree to the visibility of an assault. Press coverage is a far more powerful stimulus. The hospital is, relatively speaking, a closed world.

THE MECHANICS OF DETECTING ASSAULT

We now turn to a consideration of the mechanics of detecting assault. This is largely a matter (as police officers frequently asserted and as our case monitoring confirmed) of the availability of staunch, uncontaminated witnesses who can provide an authoritative account of the incident and clear identification of the assailant. But before examining the role of witnesses we shall consider the part played by confession evidence. Police interrogation techniques and the securing of confessions have attracted considerable criminological attention and, notwithstanding the provisions of PACE,[1] these continue to attract strong criticism (McConville *et al*. 1991: 64–75). As evidenced by the Report of the Runciman Royal Commission on Criminal Justice, this aspect of police activity remains very much under review. The fact is, however, that confessions play but a modest role in securing a guilty plea to assault or in achieving conviction at trial. This is contrary to the claim made by McConville *et al*. (1991: 57) that interrogation is '*the* central investigative strategy of the police'. A confession may provide the finishing touch to a prosecution case in respect of assault, but it is seldom, if ever, the central pillar. That at least is our view, and we shall now explain how we came to arrive at it.

For this purpose we shall consider three categories of case:

- cases in which the police have clear victim or other witness evidence in support of the charge, plus a confession;
- cases in which there is clear witness evidence but *no* confession; and
- cases in which there is questionable witness evidence and no confession.

We leave out of account those cases in which there are no witness statements and no confession: those are simply not going to be prosecuted. One may also observe from the fact that the above categorisation is built around a *second* variable, witness evidence, that we find it impossible to consider confession evidence in isolation: there is no such thing as confession evidence in the absence of an inculpating statement from the complainant or from other witnesses. Confessions, if they occur at all, are *supplementary*.

It is not our contention that because confessions are supplementary they are unimportant. This is because the police and the CPS appreciate that even apparently unequivocal identification evidence is not guaranteed to achieve conviction. The police therefore believe – and this belief informs their practice – that confession is a prize worth pursuing even where a case appears 'open and shut'. The Gerald Abbott case (31) provides one example. There were seven witness statements in this case, but the police were concerned that some of these witnesses might be reluctant to give evidence and there was also the possibility that Abbott himself might be unable to identify his assailant in an Identity Parade should one be held. Were that to have happened the prosecution case might well have collapsed. In these circumstances it is likely that a more experienced defendant would choose to say nothing. But Abbott's assailant confessed. From that point a guilty plea was assured. Another case with apparently clear-cut identification evidence was the assault upon Jonathan Musgrove (45). Here the victim had no doubt that the man he had spoken to earlier outside the pub was the person who had struck him. But the officer in the case explained that the prosecution might have difficulty in proving this. He believed that an effective defence, based on mis-identification, could have been mounted. He was surprised that the attempt was not made. These were two of several cases, many of them involving assaults in pubs or nightclubs, where what appeared from the victim's account, or from our understanding of the incident, to be a solid case based on clear identification evidence was deemed by the police to be much more fragile. Conviction *might* have been achieved without a confession. But in each case the police only became confident of the outcome once a confession was secured.

As has been said in respect of the Abbott case, a sophisticated defendant, knowing the difficulties attached to securing a conviction for assault, may choose to remain silent at police interview. Where this happens the police are of necessity thrown back on the evidence they manage to secure from the victim and other witnesses. That may or may not prove to be sufficient. In some cases – as, for example, the assaults on the two publicans, Timothy Cooper (20) and Patrick Mangan (13) – it *did* prove to be sufficient, but only because independent witnesses of good character were available in both instances. In the former case the defendant, Ray Camp, persisted in his outright denial of the charge throughout the trial. His story, backed up by a friend who was standing with him at the bar, was that he and Cooper had had an argument and that he had merely pushed Cooper in the chest, whereupon Cooper had fallen backwards on to the floor. Camp could not explain how Cooper had damaged his hand so badly, but of course it was not up to him to explain this. Conviction was secured because an independent witness, with no axe to grind, supported Cooper's version of events. But an element of doubt had been introduced into the case. The Mangan case was similar, with independent witnesses carrying the day for the prosecution. Had these witnesses not been prepared to testify, there was no guarantee that Mangan's own identification of his assailant would have been sufficient. In the words of the investigating officer: 'We would have been really struggling.'

A case in which the prosecution did indeed struggle, despite a wealth of circumstantial evidence, was the group assault upon Patrick Dashwood and his friends (3). The three more experienced defendants in this case at first declined to make statements. Subsequently they conceded peripheral involvement in the incident, but claimed that they had acted in self-defence. The police and the CPS anticipated that they would have difficulty proving the charge. They did have witnesses, but some were potentially 'hostile' while others had had only a distant view of events. In due course the defendants pleaded to a public order charge, following which the penalties imposed bore no relation to the severity of the victims' injuries. This was because it could not be established that any single defendant had been a prime mover in the incident. It might be said, therefore, that their circumspection was rewarded. Given the poor quality of the witness evidence the prosecution needed a confession, but this was denied them.

WITNESSES

It has been claimed that in any prosecution:

> [Witnesses] provide the basic structure which governs the direction of the inquiry, the selection of defendants and the choice of offence to be charged. In furnishing an advance blueprint of the shape of the evidence they enable the case to be prosecuted and defended co-herently and the trial to be supervised fairly.
>
> (Heaton-Armstrong and Wolchover 1992)

In the case of assault, certainly, it is difficult to overestimate the import-ance of witness evidence. In most of the cases which we followed it was only the availability of independent witnesses (that is to say, witnesses other than the victim) which made a prosecution viable. In fact the police took witness statements in twenty-eight of the ninety-three cases in our research sample (30 per cent). Few cases were prosecuted *without* such evidence. Respectable independent witnesses are at a premium; they are absolutely essential where the victim's own evidence might be open to question and a reassuring safety net where it is not. In the case of Cruikshank (91), a member of the Bench told us that without the independent witness the defendant might have escaped conviction. This was despite the fact that the victim was a police officer and the defendant 'a mean handbag snatcher'. The officer in the case concurred, observing that:

> He was a good witness . . . one of the magistrates had a job similar to his . . . you couldn't wish for a better man.

Most assault witnesses do not have the benefit of such respectable witnesses.

The availability of witnesses can secure conviction of marginally culpable defendants on dubious charges, just as reluctant or unreliable witnesses can imperil a case that in every other respect appears 'open and shut'. Patrick Tapnell (90) was convicted because the police had secured the evidence of two sober onlookers who had nothing to lose by assisting the police and supporting their fellow student. Compare this with the prosecution's difficulties in the case of the attack upon Dashwood and his friends. Dashwood's injuries were life-threatening, but given that the police were unable to prove who did what to whom they had little option other than to fall back on a charge of violent disorder. But the lack of credible witnesses threatened even this. As the officer in the case put it to us:

> It's witnesses. You've got to find witnesses. Because at the end of the day it says on the charge that they've caused the person on the scene to fear for his personal safety. You've got to find somebody to say: 'God, I was frightened out of my wits.' In these cases it's finding witnesses – and that's the problem we have. We'd need that even if we were charging them with assaults, because the victims basically don't remember much. It's very problematical, it really is. It's just the fact that people don't want to get involved.

The police experienced great difficulty in this case. They had to get a witness summons to secure the attendance of one 'hostile' witness at the committal stage. She was deemed to be of little value to the prosecution thereafter. Other prosecution witnesses were unavailable when the case came to trial. This led to the dropping of all assault charges and enabled the defence to argue, with some success, that their respective clients had only been on the edge of the mayhem and had done no real damage.

The Dashwood case provides one illustration of the difficulty experienced by the police in constructing a convincing account of a group assault. As the officer in the not dissimilar case of Steven Clutton (8) put it to us:

> They sound very straightforward, assaults, very ordinary, clean-cut things. But they're not. It's so complicated trying to sort out after the event when obviously the police officer wasn't there and didn't see what happened. He's got to try and build up a picture from other people and if other people are a bit anti-police they aren't going to tell you the full truth even if they did see it. So it is very difficult, very complex to piece it all together.

Witness reluctance to co-operate with the police because of general anti-police sentiment is, as suggested here, one of the reasons why the police may find it difficult to marshal an effective case. But there are also practical problems and administrative failures. For example, it is not uncommon for investigating officers to make several unavailing attempts to secure a statement from a witness over a period of weeks. This was how the principal witness to the assault on Anthony Niblett (33) recalled his experiences:

> They've asked me to make a statement. I haven't actually got together with the police officer concerned because I work shifts and so does he. So we end up working on opposite shifts. He's offered to come round to my house and take a statement but he's not pursued it any further. I said I'd go in, but that was one of the times I missed him. He'd actually gone off duty when I agreed to make a statement. So we're still waiting.

This account of missed opportunities, frustration, and lack of communication was typical of the interaction between police and witnesses which we observed.

Part of the explanation for the lack of co-operation commonly encountered by the police is the witness's reluctance to be committed to what he or she anticipates to be a tedious, frustrating process, with much hanging about at court. The assault on the pub landlord, Timothy Cooper (20), took place in a crowded pub, with fifty or sixty people present according to most estimates. But in the early stages of the investigation the officer in the case was unable to secure a statement from anyone other than Cooper and his wife. In the end, Cooper managed to locate someone who had been drinking in the pub at the time. This man was referred to by the investigating officer as an 'excellent' witness and he it was who effectively secured the conviction of the man who had 'glassed' Cooper. It is even harder to secure statements from witnesses who know the system. According to one officer, 'it's harder to convince them to make a statement than it is to get an admission out of the defendant'. The assault on Kevin Pilcher (27) was typical in this respect. The police actually asked Pilcher to gather up the five friends and acquaintances who had been with him in the pub that evening and bring them all to Central Bristol police station in order that they might make statements. According to Pilcher, none was prepared to co-operate in this enterprise.

Further to this theme of a general reluctance to become involved with the police and courts, some potential witnesses may be known to the police as offenders. This damages their credibility as witnesses but it also means that they are even less likely to want to become involved. In the case of Andrew Barker (10), the man stabbed by a taxi driver, the initial adjournment followed the non-appearance of a key witness while the final collapse of the case was the result of the victim's own failure to come to court. Both men, inhabiting the same twilight world and themselves often at odds with the police, were almost bound to prove unreliable as witnesses.

The final, most pervasive and most worrying reason for victims' and other witnesses' reluctance to assist the police is that they fear for their safety were they to do so. Even 'respectable' citizens may be reluctant to make statements because they fear retribution. For example, in the Gerald Abbott case (31) one father was not prepared to let his daughter make a statement, while neither Sally Chapman's mother nor the mother's landlord (60) were prepared to run the risk of further antagonising Chapman's assailant, Dwyer. It would have been possible for Dwyer to make both witnesses' lives intolerable, with little risk of further involvement on the part of the police. This is true over the whole spectrum of assaults, 'domestic' and otherwise: the higher up the seriousness scale the greater is police and CPS desire to secure conviction and so the more protection there is likely to be on offer, but this may still be quite limited.[2]

Some of the most severe problems of intimidation occur in relation to assaults committed within the drugs underworld. For example, the smashing up of Timothy Paxman's car and the assault on Paxman himself (6) were witnessed by several people, but the police were unable to secure a single witness statement in respect of the assault – and even Paxman went back on his own statement. It does not take a great deal of imagination to work out why. Had the landlord of Paxman's flat, where the assault took place, been prepared to 'make a complaint', then the assailant might have been charged with aggravated burglary – a very serious charge. But the landlord was unwilling even to identify the man who had assaulted Paxman, much less make his own complaint. The investigating officer was philosophical about this. He said it was unusual in the St Paul's neighbourhood for someone to interfere when they saw a person being beaten up or having their car smashed, while the police seldom obtained the co-operation of witnesses. He and his fellow officers did not feel able to be critical of this behaviour – they acknowledged that the police could not provide protection for witnesses living in the area.

The David Freeman case (4) saw a similarly determined prosecution effort following an assault by drug barons in St Paul's. In this case one witness, himself a heroin addict, did make a statement before fleeing to Manchester. Two other witnesses gave statements which were almost totally unrevealing. As it happens the police were able to locate the key independent witness on the streets of Manchester and bring him back to Bristol for the trial. Naturally they were worried about his commitment to the prosecution enterprise and, unsurprisingly, this was in due course found wanting. One of the most remarkable features of the Freeman case was the victim's own willingness to make a statement and give evidence in court, although even he was not prepared to go through this ordeal a third time. But without independent witnesses the Freeman and Paxman cases were almost bound to fail. It would have taken extraordinary courage on the part of both men, and on the part of witnesses to these very frightening events, for them to have thrown in their lot with the police. People have been killed for less.

THE POLICE, THE PROSECUTION AND THE PUBLIC

We observed many assault cases in which police officers laboured to secure statements from reluctant and elusive witnesses. Commonly they saw their labours come to nothing. In these circumstances the officers involved might be genuinely downcast, although they had typically developed psychological defences which prevented these disappointments being too crushing. The police to a considerable extent feel that they stand alone in the struggle against all forms of lawlessness, including violence (Reiner 1985: 89). As one element in this they feel locked into a hostile relationship with those defence lawyers whom the police believe adopt an antagonistic, anti-police style. The investigating officer in the David Freeman case recounted with some bitterness a conversation with a defence solicitor held in the presence of his client (who was alleged to have been one of Freeman's assailants). In the course of this conversation the solicitor observed to his client that he had been 'stitched up at the BRI (hospital) on Tuesday and stitched up at Trinity Road (police station) on Wednesday'. This remark was held to have been hostile rather than jocular, and the officer was incensed.

The police must also come to terms with sentences which they tend to regard as erring on the side of leniency. Most police officers will feel some dissatisfaction with what they regard as excessively lenient sentencing decisions (*not*, for the most part, with courts' decisions regarding guilt or innocence). They will argue that inadequate sentences make a nonsense of their own efforts to detect crime. This undermines job satisfaction and, it is implied, makes the officer less zealous in investigating all low-level crime. Officers complained to us that offenders were being given the wrong 'message' – 'I mean, he won't know where he's wrong.' They also argued that inadequate sentences were an affront to victims and, third, that they deterred victims from going to the police and from pursuing a 'complaint'. These police criticisms have some basis in reality, as our own contact with assault victims confirmed.

Despite the fact that they feel these things, officers for the most part distance themselves from the decisions of the CPS and the courts. They achieve this by adopting the rationalisation that they are but a cog in the justice machine – they need concern themselves only with their particular responsibilities, leaving the CPS and courts to discharge theirs. This was one typical observation:

> I try not to involve myself with the outcome at court actually. That's not an evasive answer, either. I generally don't bother myself with the results at court. I believe very much that my job is to gather facts and go out and do all the roles that a constable should do, and once it goes to court I feel it's the responsibility of the magistrates, the judges, and the whole of the court system to actually bring about the sentencing, or whatever decision happens.

This attitude cushions officers against disappointment, but it also limits the satisfaction available to them in dealing with routine cases. It contributes to the kind of 'uniform carrier' mentality which Reiner has noted (1985: 105) – a cynical, going through the motions approach to many tasks. We saw several examples of the limited vision of uniform officers – not surprising perhaps when they are given the task of following up a minor assault, perhaps interviewing the alleged offender but not the victim, and never discovering the final outcome. We are not surprised that officers regard this sort of thing as unrewarding labour, or that they take little interest in the case as an entity since so much of their work takes the form of connecting one nut to one bolt, rather than anything more meaningful. The fact that officers tend to distance themselves from court outcomes, not being too concerned about them, is a kind of defence mechanism which itself suggests a certain dissatisfaction with other aspects of their role. One might argue that it reflects a sense of powerlessness.

There are, as Reiner has identified, other possible police responses. One is to deliberately promote a 'tough' image, acting (as one policeman put it to us) '. . . above the public, rather than working in harmony with the public'. This is the kind of officer who, in police argot, devotes himself to 'winding people up'. But it is more common, we believe, for officers to become unenthusiastic about any case which does not offer 'easy process'. The development of a 'uniform carrier' mentality on the part of some officers may reflect their lack of personal responsibility for case conduct and perhaps also a disaffection fuelled by their experience of the court process. As a result they can display a lack of enthusiasm in pursuit of cases where there is conflicting evidence, an unsatisfactory complainant, or a lack of witnesses to hand.

We have already emphasised that even moderately experienced police officers understand the evidential demands of the court process. One must recognise, in addition, that 'constructing' a case demands a certain persistence – an investment of time and effort. Senior officers acknowledged to us that the lower ranks were on occasion disinclined to pursue problem cases. One example, cited by a Superintendent with whom we discussed this issue, concerned an assault perpetrated by a pub doorman. The victim had complained to the police and the case had been investigated. The doorman had made counter-allegations, claiming that the complainant and his friend had been causing trouble and so had had to be ejected from the pub. Faced with this conflict of evidence the investigating officer recommended that the case not be pursued, a decision endorsed by his Inspector. Subsequently the victim happened to see the Avon Chief Constable talking on television about his resolve to crack down on pub and club violence. He wrote a letter of complaint. The case was re-opened and the doorman was charged and eventually convicted of assault. It was a case which presented certain difficulties, but the eventual outcome suggests that it should not have been discontinued. Our own evidence likewise indicates that police culture favours 'cuffing' or abandonment whenever an officer believes that successful prosecution is unlikely.

It is well understood that only a very small proportion of successfully detected crime is a product of police investigative effort (Bottomley and Coleman 1980: 88f). Much detective work is purely formal. The practices of clearing up crimes by means of 't.i.c.', or by persuading a convicted offender to sign a written statement accepting responsibility for other crimes, are each well documented. These practices have obvious benefits for the police in terms of public presentation of their performance, but they have less obvious benefit for victims. Matthew Howell (49) was told by the police that they had a man in custody who had admitted to forty 'muggings' of the type suffered by Howell. They expected that this prisoner would in due course confess to robbing Howell also. Howell was unimpressed. As someone who himself lived on the margins of criminality he attributed this willingness to assign 'his' case to a known offender as evidence merely of the police failure to do their job. The investigating officer expressed some sympathy with Howell's viewpoint:

> The person that's been mugged, or whatever the crime is, at least knows that somebody's admitted doing it. But it's probably not very satisfactory from their point of view because nothing's actually done about it.

Reiner has demonstrated that 'cop culture' bears but a marginal relationship to legal rules and departmental regulations. Police practice was found to be based on 'The Ways and Means Act' and on a refusal to tolerate 'contempt of cop' (Reiner 1985: 85). Reiner argues from this that the standard response to evidence of police malpractice – slap on a new rule – may be irrelevant or even counter-productive. He also outlines what he believes to be key stages in the psychology of a typical police career, these being from *mission* to *action* to *cynicism* to *pessimism*. Both 'cuffing' and 'winding people up' reflect the policeman's inability to control the working environment or to achieve success in terms of formally approved goals. Our conversations with police officers provided plenty of evidence of the frustrations inherent in a policeman's lot. It would not be surprising if this frustration caused various forms of deviance to flourish. Perhaps unsurprisingly in a research based upon the experience of victims, the most obvious manifestation of the cynicism identified by Reiner was a lack of tenacity in pursuing difficult cases (which can be taken to include cases involving problem victims).

To summarise the main themes of this chapter, we have observed two distinct pressures on the police, reflecting two inherently problematic relationships. The first of these is with the prosecution process and the court; the second is with the public. One needs to be aware of the pains and dissatisfactions, from the police perspective, inherent in both these relationships in order to understand the way the police act. It has been suggested (Bottomley and Coleman 1980: 94) that public debate about crime and the police should be switched to an examination of the objectives of policing and public expectations of the police – this with a view to improving 'the quality and quantity of police/citizen interaction' so as to achieve 'a shared responsibility for law and order'. Police contact with suspects does not always take place in the controlled environment of the police station, where it may be assumed that the police are in an overwhelmingly powerful position, the suspect in a very vulnerable one. Many street encounters can be extremely painful for the police, involving high levels of stress. This is a product of the aggressively anti-police attitude of many young working-class males, both black and white. Night shifts are especially harrowing. PC Pratt (28), who figures in our sample as a victim, told of being called in the early hours to a city centre multi-storey car park where 20 or 30 cars were racing one another. If the officer attempted to talk to one of these 'boy racers' he would find himself surrounded by a large group of them. There would then be concerted verbal abuse of the officer, coupled with physical intimidation:

> They'll try to stare you out . . . rub noses with you . . . push up against you until your helmet goes back and you're literally forehead to forehead. And you've just got to push people away, or say: 'If you don't go, you're gonna be arrested.'

One factor which influences the police response to this kind of baiting is their understanding that it would be virtually impossible successfully to prosecute any of those involved – in which case there might seem little point in making an arrest. It is apparent from this kind of account that young policemen face a great many encounters from which they struggle to escape without loss of face. The risk of 'image loss' is as much a factor for policemen as it is for the young men they are called upon to control. Typically the officer will attempt in these circumstances to deliver himself of a speech indicating the likely costs of persisting in such behaviour. But he or she may well fear that such a response is inadequate. In short, the officer is likely to feel damaged by the encounter.

In relation to known offenders whom the police frequently arrest, there is, in contrast, a premium upon maintaining cordial relations. Detectives, especially, pride themselves on their ability to get on well with their 'customers'. For example, the officer investigating the David Freeman assault considered that he had a good relationship with most of the gang who had kidnapped Freeman. There was no need to be unpleasant, was his view. Other detectives echoed this. They held that if they treated defendants decently it made their job easier. The object, said one detective, was to conduct the interview in an atmosphere such that, if you were to meet that person again, you would be able to have a joke and a chat. The detective constable who interviewed the assailant in the Duke case (69) complained that he found him 'a strange fellow to deal with' because he was not prepared to offer any explanation as to why he had assaulted the two young women. The officer was frustrated at being denied not just an admission, but any meaningful exchange with the defendant. This, we would argue, is part of any police officer's job satisfaction, independent of his securing conviction. Most feel a need to maintain a good relationship with their local community, including the 'community' of habitual offenders.

Where a particular district presents special problems, as does St Paul's in Bristol, officers take pride in their ability to penetrate local *mores*. St Paul's has a mixed race population, with a large African–Caribbean element. It is commonly asserted that police officers are hostile or at least suspicious in their dealings with blacks (Reiner 1985: 100). The police, it is said, regard blacks as especially prone to crime, and as volatile and hard to handle. Reiner's own research involved interviews with police officers in St Paul's in 1973/4. He found that 35 per cent of police in the Central division of Bristol (including St Paul's) volunteered adverse comments about blacks. Our own discussions with officers, both in St Paul's and in other areas of the city, reveal that their attitude towards blacks is more subtle and complex than might be inferred from studies carried out prior to the riots of 1982. Police culture may have changed in the last 15 to 20 years. That is not to deny that there is prejudice, of course, but there are also signs of a reasonable working relationship reflecting a measure of tolerance. For the most part the St Paul's police officers with whom we discussed these matters claimed to get on well with black people and said they also managed to relate, on a professional basis, to black criminals. One officer boasted of how he had managed to create a favourable impression through his grasp of some of the *patois*. Another, the officer in the Macintosh case (66), likewise took pride in his ability to get along with black suspects. The interview which he had conducted with the defendant in this case did not present insuperable problems:

Basically, I got on with him fine. He's the sort of person you can talk to, who will talk, will give you information, and will tell you partly the truth. He's not hostile to the police. He was OK – no problem at all. He said: 'I know I done wrong – I lost my temper.'

The picture we describe is consistent with Policy Studies Institute research (1993, Vol. IV: 109) which found a mixture of racist attitudes among the police and yet predominantly good relations with most black suspects. This is rather remarkable given that, as Reiner points out, societal racism places ethnic minorities disproportionately in those strata from which the police derive their 'property' (Reiner 1985: 81). Nonetheless it is consistent with the picture, which we believe is accurate, of the police making some effort to modify their image as an oppressive 'force' preying on certain sections of the community. The police have to deal with the public on a day-to-day basis, just as they have to deal with the CPS and the courts. To present them as able to manipulate these two sets of relationships to their own organisational ends is an over-simplification. The police are manipulative in the service of their own interests, as is any other organisational group, but they are not in an especially strong position. They have to *persuade* the CPS and *persuade* the courts. Perhaps it is because they struggle to exert influence in the legal arena that the police have resolved to accentuate the positive side of their relationship with complainants and suspects.

Chapter 6

Police case construction

When an assault is reported and judged worthy of investigation it may give rise to an arrest. The assault then becomes a 'case' and all its constituent elements will be contained within a file destined for the CPS. The transformation of an incident, allegedly of assault, into a case file involves a process of selection and interpretation. McConville *et al.* (1991: 11) refer to this process as one of 'case construction'. We do not object to that description and indeed we adopt it, as reflecting the processes of interpretation, translation, consolidation and limitation by which an event as complicated as an assault is packaged to enable it to be presented to a court. It is beyond question, as we shall demonstrate, that the prosecution case does indeed have to be 'constructed': the case file is never merely an assembly of all the relevant facts. In this respect it is difficult to take seriously the view advanced by the Runciman Royal Commission on Criminal Justice (Chapter 5, para. 2), namely:

> We see as central to [the relationship between police and CPS] the unambiguous separation of the role of investigator and prosecutor. . . . In our view, just as the police should concentrate on discovering the facts relevant to an alleged or reported criminal offence, including those which may tend to exonerate the suspect, so should the CPS concentrate on assessing both the strengths and weaknesses of the case which, if the decision is taken to proceed, will bring the defendant before the courts.

In other words, the Royal Commission was not prepared to acknowledge that there is such a thing as police case construction. Such a view cannot be sustained in the face of the available research evidence.

We would also concur with the view of McConville *et al.* (1991: 203) that the prosecution case cannot be seen to reflect disagreement or confusion. Doubts and uncertainties, or competing versions of events, will of course be asserted by the *defence*, but these cannot be accepted by the prosecution because the prosecution objective is to prove the charge. Different interpretations, perhaps reflecting the complication of a prior personal relationship between victim and defendant, will, of necessity, be played down by the prosecution. It is not the job of the prosecution to introduce competing versions of 'what really happened'; that is for the defence. The case for the prosecution will contain a single, coherent account of the incident in question. The process of case construction is designed – inevitably so, given the adversarial presumption upon which criminal justice operates – to assert this unitary view.[1]

In this chapter we shall describe the process of police case construction in respect of assault, but without replicating the image of all-embracing police power which is presented by McConville and his co-authors. They focus unremittingly upon the construction of criminality; they appear uninterested in, or attach little importance to, the construction of *non-criminality* (Boyle 1993). As far as McConville *et al.* are concerned, weak cases are simply weak cases – and weak cases should not be pursued. They appear not to be interested in *why* a case is weak. They acknowledge that case construction cuts both ways, but the only construction that really interests them is the construction of guilt. Theirs is a partial view.

Our monitoring of assault cases revealed that the processes of interpretation and case construction begin with the police officer's initial contact with a potential complainant. The initial police interpretation may seriously prejudice any subsequent investigation. Take, for example, the assault on Michael Fleming (7). Fleming was struck on the head with a brick while driving through St Paul's. He had earlier been involved in an altercation with a motorist (and his passenger) whose route he had blocked while seeking to attach a broken-down vehicle to his trailer truck. Fleming suffered a multiple skull fracture but managed to get out of his vehicle and was walking around, covered in blood, when the police arrived. He was incoherent and may well have been behaving in what appeared a belligerent or threatening fashion. It is tempting to speculate that the police viewed him as a control problem and were concerned that this 'disturbance' be dealt with as speedily as possible. This perception may have been encouraged by the fact that the incident took place on what is generally regarded as the most dangerous street in Bristol from the police point of view (and indeed from the point of view of any chance passer-by). It was perhaps because of this that the police failed to grasp both the extent of Fleming's injury and the background to the assault. As a result of the police mis-reading, no crime report was filed although the incident was 'logged' on the record of the police vehicle's activities for the evening in question. The log read that 'the injured party refused to make a complaint'. It is a bit much, one might think, to be deemed not to have made a complaint when you are suffering the immediate aftermath of what was described to the victim as one of the worst skull fractures ever to be brought to the Bristol Royal Infirmary. It would have been far better for Fleming had he been rendered unconscious. It is of course difficult for us to tell how much Fleming's appearance (a long-haired, heavily built biker) and the location of the incident contributed to this misinterpretation. Perhaps the police would have been more alert to other possibilities had they seen a soberly suited individual in a similarly blood-soaked state on a street in Clifton. Speaking personally, one hopes so.

The subsequent police 'construction', when an investigation did at last get under way, appeared designed to downplay the incident and was perhaps a retrospective justification for their initial lacklustre response. In the words of the investigating officer:

> From the investigations which we carried out I don't think that the brick was in fact thrown at *him*. I think it was thrown at his truck, and he was unlucky in the way it hit him.

Now this was at odds with Michael Fleming's own account. He was adamant that the brick had been brought crashing down on his head. This, although we are not medically qualified to judge, seems more consistent with the injuries which he suffered than does the police account. It is tempting, therefore, to regard the police account as something of a rationalisation – the version which they would *prefer* to believe. Of course we cannot be sure that Fleming's account was accurate – but nor can we see any justification for the police view of the matter being expressed as forthrightly as it was by the investigating officer – particularly given that, as he admitted to us, he had been told several different versions of what had occurred. He said at one point:

> There is nobody who actually saw the actual incident. There are people who saw what was going to happen, and people who saw after it happened, but nobody saw the whole thing in its entirety.

So how could he be certain that the brick was thrown rather than smashed down on Fleming's head, and how could he be certain that it was thrown at the truck and not at Fleming?

Questions of interpretation arose overtly at the outset of several other cases. Matthew Collins (35) perceived himself as a victim, and seemed to have a reasonable case for doing so:

> He ran at me. There was a window behind me. He done a rugby tackle. I seen a piece of glass come down towards my face so I put my hand up to save my face.

As a result of this attack Collins suffered a severe injury to his hand. He also found himself in court accused of a public order offence and criminal damage, on level terms with his attacker. His perception of what had happened was entirely at odds with that of the officer who came to the scene and who regarded the only true 'victim' as the shopkeeper whose window had been broken. The gap between the two perceptions is reflected in Collins' observation:

> I felt they were getting carried away. I felt like a train robber when I was, you know, a bloke who got pushed through a window.

Although Collins' assailant was initially charged with ABH, the police gave the impression that they viewed the two men in much the same light – that is, as having posed a common threat to public order. The CPS directed that the assault charge be dropped so that, rightly or wrongly, Collins' status as 'victim' disappeared from the script and he was presented to the court, unambiguously, as an offender. Thus the officer's initial judgement of what had happened, arrived at in the absence of any witness statements, determined the way in which the case would be framed thereafter. He formed the view, having talked to the two men, that both were culpable. We suspect that the assault charge (to which the officer was never strongly committed) was dropped by the CPS because it might have been thought inconsistent with the prosecution claim that Collins had deliberately smashed the window rather than having been pushed backwards through it.

It is quite common for the police to be met by the chaotic aftermath of a violent confrontation which they must then try to piece together. A typical police response in these circumstances is to seek to identify the offender from among those still present at the scene – that is to say, there is a tendency to target an identifiable suspect, even if that person is a somewhat implausible assailant by virtue of being, say, a friend of the victim or someone who claims 'victim' status on his or her own account. The police are not always deterred from making an arrest even in circumstances where their suspicions appear to be convincingly rebutted. This was the pattern in the case of Andrew Barker (10), who was stabbed in the leg and chest following a drunken argument with a taxi-driver.

When the police arrived they arrested Barker's friend, Tommy, who is black, and Sandy, the girl with whom he had attempted to get into the taxi. Sandy and Tommy were both kept in police cells overnight although Tommy had not been involved in the incident at all. One can see the need for immediate action by the police – at least then they do not have to go on looking for a suspect; but it is obviously unsatisfactory if this instant response is made on the basis of inaccurate information. Tommy was released after 16 hours in custody and the police eventually arrested the taxi-driver, who had left the scene before they arrived. We noted a similar pattern following the assault upon Nigel Jenks (30) in Bristol city centre. Jenks was attacked from behind with a heavy object and rendered unconscious, suffering a broken cheekbone. He never saw his assailant. In this case the police arrested two men who had been involved in a nearby altercation, one of them a member of the group which included Jenks. They then accused the men whom they had arrested of attacking Jenks. The victim regarded the suggestion that his friend had assaulted him as utterly preposterous.

This then is a persistent theme – the police tend to work on whoever it is they have to hand. This may in part be a reflection of a 'tidy mind' mentality, with the police seeking to tie up all the loose ends in relation to whoever it is they have in custody. But it also suggests that decisions made by officers who are first on the scene may be crucial in determining what happens thereafter. In so far as there was any detective work done in the Jenks case, it seemed almost to be a matter of pinning whichever crimes had been committed that evening upon the inhabitants of the cells in Bristol Central police station. In summary, there is a tendency for police case construction to follow the path of least resistance – or at least, of ready availability. The most extreme example of this which we observed involved the arrest of an alleged assault victim, John Enwright (39), on the basis that the 'assault' was a cover for a robbery. Enwright was a former police officer. This was his version of events:

> When those guys nicked me there, I just felt that they were – for the sake of a statistic – picking me out because it was an easy option. They had nobody – they had no suspect. So they just turned it round their way. It's the old routine: you've got nothing to lose, you give the guy a hard time – who knows, he may cough to it in the end anyway, whether he's done it or not. If he does, you've struck lucky; if not, you just let him go. All you've done is inconvenience him a bit. There's less paperwork for them.

Of course the officers in this case may have had experience of other fabricated assaults which were designed to enable a robber to get away with a crime. We cannot say that the police were mistaken in this case, but it is noteworthy that they had not questioned anybody else in connection with the robbery other than the manager at the depot where the victim/suspect worked. In part perhaps this was because the police could not devote much manpower to following up one rather unpromising robbery. But there was also the fact that they had decided in their own minds that the alleged 'victim' was guilty, and since they believed that they would never secure a conviction unless he were to admit the matter they saw little point in pursuing other lines of enquiry which presupposed an alternative robber in whom they themselves did not believe. It is the fact of their imposing this interpretation upon events which is of interest to us – that and their reluctance to give credence to the 'victim''s account.

The same detective was, as it happens, involved in each of three investigations alluded to above:

- the assault on Nigel Jenks in the city centre;
- the stabbing of Andrew Barker; and
- the burglary and 'assault' upon John Enwright at the weighbridge.

The detective's approach in each instance was paradoxical in that he sought to apprehend either the victim himself or a friend of the victim. The question arises: is this simply a feature of this officer's technique, perhaps based on his experience of other cases of this kind, or is it a lazy detective-constable's way of following the only avenue which he sees opening up before him? Whichever explanation one believes, this rather bizarre pattern gives us some insight into the difficulty of detecting 'stranger' assaults. It also gives an indication of the problems posed for the police by a lack of truly innocent victims or of indisputably culpable offenders. It is unsurprising, given the need to establish manifest culpability and (relative) innocence for the purposes of criminal prosecution, that the absence of these characteristics can lead to dubious or even manifestly erroneous 'constructions'.

Suspected lack of innocence may deter police action even where the alleged victim (that is to say, the complainant) has suffered serious injury. This is typical of assaults involving young men. For example, there is a history of gang warfare between groups of youths from various outlying districts of Bristol. Anthony Glover (42) went to the police, claiming that he had been assaulted by youths from a neighbouring village whom he had met by chance. His jaw had been broken. But the officer on whose 'patch' the incident occurred was disinclined to take the matter further. He believed that the meeting was pre-arranged. As he explained to us:

> If somebody goes in a drunken state looking for a fight then I think the majority of people, policemen or otherwise, would say: 'You've got the beating, boy, and you asked for it. If you didn't go there looking for it, you wouldn't have found it.'

He also said of the victim: 'If he'd been an innocent party, he'd have rung me back again.' In other words, the victim's lack of innocence was inferred from his having consumed a large quantity of alcohol and from his lack of persistence in pursuing his 'complaint' when met with initial police scepticism. Of course the scepticism may have been justified, but it is the construction which is of interest to us – that and the fact that this construction may go either way; it may be inculpatory or exculpatory.

In some instances police case construction reflects their prior knowledge of both victim and assailant. In the case of the assault upon William Kenny (43) in a pub car-park in Wells the investigating officer told us that one of his colleagues knew the alleged assailant and that 'he was not the type to use a weapon with which to hit somebody'. This estimation carried some weight with the officer – it formed part of the picture which he had built up of the injured man being at least as much sinning as sinned against. He believed that Kenny's injuries had been suffered as he fell, his head striking the ground. Kenny for his part claimed that his assailant had been a school friend of some of the police officers and even now was a member of the same rugby club. It is unsurprising, this assault having taken place in a small town, that the various actors should display some knowledge of one another. The police assessment reflected their understanding of the local scene in which Kenny and his assailant were known characters. They based their interpretation of what had taken place on this prior knowledge as much as they did on the various witness statements. Nonetheless, despite their reservations, the police made an arrest, a s. 20 GBH charge was preferred, and a conviction was obtained on that count. The police would say that despite their entertaining some scepticism about Kenny the evidence was there and so they were bound to act upon it.

Nonetheless it is fair to say that the victim's story is likely to be *tested* by initial police scepticism; in Kenny's case the story survived. But there can also be other tests. The most common, and most demanding, is the emergence of alternative stories – whether supplied by the alleged assailant or by witnesses. It is in the nature of assault that there will tend to be competing accounts of the incident, these accounts being incompatible with one another. The police will sometimes say, particularly with reference to violent incidents involving young men, that the 'victim' is the person who first arrives at the police station. Such a view of assault is itself a construction, and an overly cynical one. However the fact remains that it is difficult for a third party, not present at the scene, to assign blame. This can be illustrated by the case of Ann Parkinson (67) who got into an argument with her (female) flat-mate and who was then struck several times by the flat-mate's father. She presented herself to us, and to the police, as a hapless victim. The flat-mate and her parents had a very different story to tell: they claimed that the aggression had stemmed from Parkinson, she having attacked both mother and daughter. The outraged husband/father had then come to the rescue of his 'womenfolk'. As commonly happens following an allegation of assault, Parkinson's three adversaries made counter-allegations against her and asked the police to act on those. The case was referred to the CPS but they were unimpressed by both sets of complainants and discontinued the case. The police regarded the incident as essentially 'domestic' – this itself being a construction with its own implicit case management prescription.

Some cases are strong enough to withstand the impact of these alternative stories: they have other positive features which, together, convince the police and the CPS that they should see the business through. One such was the assault on the retired policeman, Gerald Abbott (31). A new slant was given to this assault when several witnesses indicated that Abbott had been the instigator in the limited sense that he had intervened in a public argument between a youth and his girlfriend. The officer in the case accepted this somewhat modified version of events. He said to us:

Had [Abbott] not intervened, and just walked past, he wouldn't have been assaulted, without a shadow of a doubt.

So this was the construction which this officer placed on these events. It did not make him any less zealous in pursuing the investigation, as one might expect given that this was a nasty assault perpetrated by a 19 year old, possessor of an extensive criminal record, upon a 59-year-old retired policeman. Nonetheless the 'provocation', such as it was, doubtless figured in the case papers and this may have been a factor in the subsequent CPS decision to downgrade the charge to one of s. 47.

POLICE PERCEPTION OF THE ASSAILANT

It has been suggested that an officer's negative feelings towards a suspect may lead him or her to upgrade that person's criminality, as in declining to caution where a caution would have been appropriate (McConville *et al*. 1991: 59). Conversely, the same researchers noted a police 'sense of fairness' in cases where their sympathies lay with the offender, leading them to charge at a low level and to incorporate elements of mitigation into the case papers (*ibid*.: 104). Our own research findings support this. An assailant who is obstructive towards officers, or who goes so far as to assault them following an attack on a member of the public, is likely to be dealt with severely. This is especially true where the offender has a prior criminal record. The young man who attacked Louise Duke (69) had several previous convictions for burglary. In perpetrating a relatively minor assault upon Duke and her friend he initiated a chain of events which culminated in his being sentenced to 12 months' imprisonment. Whenever there was this clear-cut ascription of roles – wholly innocent victim; clearly culpable and belligerent offender – it contributed to officers' determination to press ahead with the case.

Conversely, where the assailant is not drunk, displays no 'contempt of cop', and his dress and general demeanour suggested an upright citizen, the police are likely to respond with a certain sympathy. This was evident in the case of Peter White (25), the young man who with a single blow broke the jaw of Edward Jones following a motoring dispute. The officer in the case regarded White as having been unfortunate to find himself charged with a criminal offence: as a young white-collar worker and university graduate he was not a typical offender. Despite the fact that White (possibly rather ill-advisedly) pleaded not guilty, his readiness to co-operate with the police was confirmed in court by the officer. This is not uncommon: police perceptions of the offender influence the subsequent presentation of the case. That said, the police are unlikely to drop the case altogether, although we did come across one instance – the group assault upon Patrick Dashwood and his friends (3) – where charges were dropped in respect of one of the accused in the course of a complex plea-bargaining operation. This man was, arguably, the instigator of the attack, but the investigating officer was quite sympathetic towards him, referring to him as 'quite a nice man . . . he comes from a different background'. The fact that this one defendant played the game by the officer's rules and generally impressed him as a reasonable fellow *may* have been a factor in his being allowed to walk free from the court, although of course this was a CPS decision at this stage. Nonetheless police perceptions of the defendants may have fed through into the plea-bargaining process just as they feed through into the prosecutor's presentation of the case in court.

Occasionally, in keeping with the paradoxical investigative reasoning to which reference has already been made, we observed a cross-over of police allegiance from victim to offender, as in the assault upon Andrew Barker (10). When we interviewed the investigating officer in this case the first thing he said to us was:

> By their own admission Andrew Barker and the young lady he was in company with had been out drinking quite heavily throughout the day. There is no doubt that they were extremely drunk.

Even after the police had concluded that Barker had been knifed by the taxi-driver, the officer's sympathies clearly lay with the taxi-driver and he appeared to accept his version of events in so far as it was possible for him to do so. Barker's status as victim was compromised by his criminal record and by the company he kept. As the officer explained, the public house where Barker had been drinking on the night he was stabbed was a notorious venue for drug dealing.

But it is important to acknowledge that even in the Barker case there was no evidence that an unfavourable police perception of the victim and a favourable impression of the alleged assailant made a significant difference to police processing of the case. In other words, police assessments of the character of victim and assailant, taken in isolation, have but limited impact upon case construction. The arresting officer in the Barker case, while he had little sympathy with the victim, observed that he was 'no less entitled to be believed than a witness of previous good character'. While one might be inclined to take this particular observation with a pinch of salt, the evidence of our research is that these police judgements do not influence their decision-making where they have a clear-cut offence, a readily identifiable assailant, and a staunch complainant.

THE SIGNIFICANCE OF THE ASSAILANT'S RACE

Our data suggest that black assailants run a *lower* risk of detection and prosecution than do whites. Among our sample of ninety-three cases there were twenty successful prosecutions of white assailants out of sixty-one cases (33 per cent); and two successful prosecutions of black assailants out of twenty-four cases (8 per cent). This is not explained by a difference in the rate of reporting: reporting rates were broadly comparable in respect of black and white assailants. But cases involving black assailants were less likely to be detected by the police. Also, a higher proportion of cases involving black defendants saw the victim decline to co-operate with the prosecution at court. In respect of the sixty-one white assailants whose cases we followed, there was no court hearing in thirty-seven cases (61 per cent); three cases were dismissed (5 per cent); there were seventeen guilty pleas (26 per cent); three convictions were achieved following trial (7 per cent); and there was one not guilty finding (2 per cent). In respect of the twenty-four black assailants, there was no court hearing in eighteen cases (78 per cent); four cases were dismissed (17 per cent); and there were two guilty pleas (8 per cent).

Those black suspects who were charged tended to face more serious charges than did whites. Of the six blacks who were charged, one was charged initially with s. 47 assault and the other five (83 per cent) were charged with s. 18 GBH. Of the twenty-four whites who were charged, one (4 per cent) was charged with a public order offence, ten (42 per cent) were initially charged with a s. 47 assault, eight (33 per cent) were charged with s. 20 assault, and five (21 per cent) were charged with s. 18 assault (including one also charged with rape). This pattern could be attributed to one (or more) of the following:

- there is police racism in 'charging up' black assailants;
- blacks do indeed commit more serious violence;
- low level assaults perpetrated by blacks are less likely to be reported than are equivalent assaults perpetrated by whites; or
- the police tend to detect only the most serious assaults perpetrated by blacks whereas they have more success across the board in detecting assaults by whites.

Our case analysis reveals the latter two explanations to be nearer the mark, this in turn being a reflection of the particular circumstances of these assaults, and also of the areas in which the offences took place. In summary, a higher proportion of assaults perpetrated by blacks were 'stranger' assaults, while of those cases in which victim and assailant were known to one another, a higher proportion of victims assaulted by blacks appeared unwilling to go to the police.

THE IMPOSITION OF POLICE VIEWS IN STATEMENT-TAKING

Under the provisions of the Police and Criminal Evidence Act 1984 interviews with suspects are tape-recorded and a summary transcription made. But interviews with witnesses (including the victim) are still written out by hand. To date the main focus of judicial and academic interest has been the interview with the suspect: it has been suggested, for example, that these interrogations involve putting the police version of events to the suspect, rather than eliciting the suspect's version (McConville *et al.* 1991: 77). We regard the preparation of *witness* statements as equally problematic. Several of the victims whose cases we followed considered that the process of recording their statement had involved editing and transforming their account so that it might better meet the demands of the prosecution process. The process of statement-taking can be seen as the first step in the victim's progressive alienation from his or her 'story' by the processes of the law. This is so even where the victim is treated with some delicacy by the police. Miranda Hooper (1), a rape victim, accepted that the investigating officers had done almost everything in their power to assist her, but one thing they appeared *not* prepared to do was to take down her statement verbatim. Since the events she described had taken place over a long period her account was necessarily lengthy and the process of taking it down long-hand was laborious. Hooper, an educated and articulate person, identified the way in which the resulting statement was at one remove from her experience:

> It was my statement put in her language, which felt quite odd. . . . She wrote it out and she had to do a few amendments. But one can't be too pernickety about it, so I left a few things which were not exactly inaccurate but weren't exactly how I would have put it.

Anthony Niblett (33), a homosexual assaulted by another gay man, told us that he would have welcomed the chance to amend his original statement in order to include in it details which, on reflection, he considered material to the incident. These details, he said, would have conveyed more of the context of the assault:

> I'd want to make it a bit clearer. There are things I haven't said that should be said. I'd been subjected to things for quite a few weeks before it actually happened. I think that's important, that it ought to be put down. That I had not, you know, reacted to provocation for a long time.

Niblett's wish to give a fuller statement reflected his sense that the criminalisation process ought to be able to respond to the broad context of a single act of violence. But the police tend not to record what the *victim* considers to be significant context-setting material.

Where an interviewee's status is in doubt, with the police perhaps preferring an alternative construction under which the victim is transformed into an offender, the statement-taking process becomes, inevitably, much less sympathetic, with words and meanings being altered to a point where they become quite at odds with what the victim (that is to say, the person claiming to have been victimised) intended. McConville *et al.* (1991: 56–79) provide transcript evidence of the way in which officers create 'legitimate' facts as a result of their acceptance or rejection of accounts preferred by victims or defendants. Once these facts are established on file the case begins to harden, with the result that there may be no opportunity to challenge the prosecution version of events. This is borne out by the case of Matthew Collins (35). Collins, who had no previous experience of the police, claimed that he was not permitted to say what he wanted to say in interview. He was ready to admit that he had been verbally aggressive, but he wished to deny that he had at any stage contributed to the violence:

> When I done the statement . . . I reckoned it was all wrong. 'Cos they just put their side of it. I said 'Leave the fighting out of it', and he said 'Well, if there wasn't any fighting, you wouldn't have gone through the window.' I explained to him about ten times there wasn't any fighting, I just got pushed. And he was going 'Well, that ain't my problem, mate, you've just got to prove that in court haven't you?' Well, I think that's well out of order.

Collins felt that the police were unprepared to accept – or to *record* – his version of how he had come by his injuries. In the end he signed a statement which he believed misrepresented what had happened. He agreed to pay an equal share of compensation for the damage to the window, but he continued to protest his innocence:

> I just want to get it over with, basically. In court I ain't really bothered if I win or lose; I just want to get it over and out of the way.

If one were to believe Collins – and we believed him – he was a victim of criminal processing as much as he was a victim of his assailant.

The changes to their story experienced by other, less controversial victims was much less stark, but their statements as written might nonetheless be selective and marginally inaccurate versions of what they had dictated. This is a theme developed by Heaton-Armstrong and Wolchover (1992), who claim 'a strong motivation [on the part of the police] to control the content of civilian witness statements'. These authors refer in passing to reluctance by the CPS and police to release details of initial complaints by witnesses as recorded on crime reports, the insinuation being that the publication of such information would threaten police control of witness statements and the solidity of the prosecution case.

We should pause here because we are in danger of falling in with – and indeed perpetuating – an image of police investigation as all-powerful, or at least *effective* in 'constructing' a water-tight prosecution case. This, in our view, is a misrepresentation. The police do indeed strive to construct a strong case, and their reluctance to permit witnesses to draft their own statements can be understood in this light, but assault, perhaps above all other offences, presents problems of interpretation with regard to the allocation of responsibility and blame. The police are reluctant to construct a case which, while it might be effective in prosecution terms, would in their view misrepresent the balance of culpability. They have their own code of values – a code which transcends questions of legal guilt or innocence (Reiner 1985: 94–7). That said, the police have to arrive at a coherent and persuasive account of a disputed event which they themselves did not witness. This does call for a process of case construction, but this construction need not be as goal-oriented as presented by McConville *et al*. The police have to arrive at a 'story', but this story may fail to reflect the gravity of an offence just as much as it may embellish it. Many assault victims whom we interviewed alleged the former. This partly reflected the inevitable need to arrive at an *interpretation* in response to an allegation of assault, and partly, on occasion, it reflected a failure to marshall the available evidence, perhaps because insufficient time and effort had been devoted to the task. One example of this second phenomenon concerned the assault upon an off-duty policeman, Jonathan Musgrove (45). The victim in this case was strongly critical of the way in which the investigating officer had failed to include medical evidence, a failure which, as he saw it, prevented his case being properly presented in court:

> To cut a long story short, his solicitor stood up and said 'Yes, my client fully admitted an assault on this gentleman and hitting him to the ground.' The local police had not included photographs of my injuries, they'd not made any attempt to include a dental report, to include a medical report (which obviously would have shown the injuries I got: broken nose, broken jaw, broken tooth, the lips, the lot), and basically the CPS said 'Yes, fine, he's pleading guilty to the assault' and he was fined £150.

So the police file, as Musgrove saw it, inadequately represented the harm done to him. The investigating officer, on the other hand, suggested that Musgrove's injuries, though serious, were not of the scale which he implied. This was a fairly typical conflict between victim and police perceptions. Musgrove himself was sufficiently aggrieved to initiate an investigation into the conduct of his case. It goes without saying that a lay victim, believing a case to be inadequately presented, would be much less likely to be able to identify the cause of this inadequacy or to be in a position to initiate an investigation. The Musgrove case underlines the importance of 'paperwork' in case construction, a point made with some force by McConville *et al.* As the case progresses the gathered statements, including the statements of 'experts', such as doctors, do indeed become *the case*. It is the material contained in this prosecution file, a 'construction' which may reflect diminution or embellishment, which largely determines the conduct of the case thereafter, including the court's sentence, if there is to be a sentence.

DETERMINING THE CHARGE

One obvious product of police case construction, in the sense we use this term, is the initial charge. In the case of assault there is a fine gradation from s. 39 ('common assault') through to s. 18 ('grievous bodily harm with intent'). The different levels of charge are supposed to reflect intent and the nature of the injury suffered. The truth is that the different levels of charge are essential elements in the smooth *administration* of criminal justice and function, in effect, as bargaining counters within a plea-bargaining system. But the initial charge does, very roughly, correspond to the police view of the seriousness of the assault. The breakdown of initial charges among the ninety-three cases which we followed is given in Table 6.1 below. In fact thirty-one cases out of ninety-three gave rise to a criminal charge. The charges first put by the police comprise roughly equal numbers of s. 47, s. 20 and s. 18 counts. There were *no* s. 39 ('common assault') charges at this stage.

The definition of harm in relation to s. 47 and s. 20 charges is such that some quite serious attacks may, as a result of the type of injuries caused, fall into the lower category. A police officer explained how unsatisfactory he felt the distinction between the two charges to be:

> It's always been a bit of an anomaly to me because you can have quite a minor cut but because the skin is broken it's classified as a wounding, but you can have quite serious bruising over a lot of your body and really considerable discomfort, far more than you get from a small cut, and you [the assailant] are going to be charged with ABH.

Table 6.1 The charge first put

Police not informed	18(19.4%)
No charge	44(47.3%)
Section 47	11(11.8%)
Section 20 GBH	8(8.6%)
Section 18 GBH	11(11.8%)
Public Order Offence (only)	1(1.1%)
Total	93(100%)

Although both s. 47 and s. 20 carry a maximum penalty of five years' imprisonment, the perception remains that ABH is the lesser charge (a defendant charged with s. 20 assault is more likely to have his or her case refused summary trial, while punishments for ABH tend to be lower than for GBH).

In some cases the charge reflected not only the nature of the injuries but also the officer's assessment of the assailant's motivation and his or her view of the circumstances surrounding the incident – in other words, of the offender's culpability in the broadest sense. Matthew Saunders (2) was blinded in one eye when an umbrella was thrown at him, spear fashion, through the glass panel of his front door. The investigating officer decided to charge the assailant, Michael Addis, who was well known to Saunders, with s. 20 assault rather than with s. 18. The officer, who charged Addis without first speaking to Saunders, readily accepted Addis' claim that he had not intended to injure Saunders as severely as in fact he had. The s. 20 charge reflected the officer's understanding that the assault had been an unfortunate accident. He told us that Addis could hardly be thought to have aimed at Saunders' eye: the s. 20 charge – wounding without intent – reflected this. The officer may also have been influenced by the fact that this assault had certain elements of the 'domestic', with both Saunders and Addis being involved with the one woman. This perhaps explains why, despite the gravity of Saunders' injuries, the investigating officer had contemplated not bringing *any* charges against Addis.

So the Saunders case once more confirms the importance of the initial police interpretation and weighing of the evidence. From the perspective of the victim this was very much an under-construction: Saunders was bitterly aggrieved at the level of charge, as the investigating officer confirmed. It appeared to Saunders, and to us, that this reflected a police presumption in favour of his assailant. It is arguable that the seeds of the eventual not guilty verdict were contained within this initial police decision: at the trial the defence was able to argue that Addis should be acquitted because (among other things) the decision to charge him with a s. 20 assault rather than s. 18 indicated that the prosecution must have been aware that they would be unable to prove intent.

This supports the contention of McConville *et al.* (1991: 141–7) that the CPS are generally not in a position to challenge police case construction, including police assessment of seriousness. Nonetheless the police are *not* all-powerful. The police approach to framing the initial charge in cases of assault serves to illustrate this. The police have no control over the charge *eventually* put, and they feel this limitation keenly. Their decisions concerning the initial charge are to a degree tactical, taken in the expectation of a downward revision of the charge by the CPS. The police *expect* that the CPS will be prepared to offer a revised charge in return for a guilty plea. With this in mind officers may put the initial charge up a notch in anticipation of its being plea-bargained down. We saw an instance of this when the defendants in the Dashwood case (3) were charged with s. 18 assaults although solid evidence against them was hard to find. In the end the CPS accepted guilty pleas to violent disorder. The investigating officer in the case of Louise Duke (69) admitted that the assailant had been charged with s. 20 assault on the arresting police officers (one of whom broke a thumb) because it was felt that such a charge would 'show his criminality' and because 'it gives the CPS leeway to reduce the charges to s. 47 assaults'. Does this suggest a manipulative, all-powerful police? Manipulative certainly, but this is in response to the limitations upon the exercise of police power which flow from the fact that the police must submit, without question, to the authority of the CPS.

Police officers recognise that the final decision concerning the charge rests with the CPS, as does any further reduction or dropping of charges in the course of last minute plea-bargaining. Police officers are jealous of their own authority, but they have come to terms with CPS control over the prosecution process, including the CPS role in determining the charge. They define their own role accordingly. That is not to say that officers *welcome* the imposition of CPS judgements. Some express resentment, a fairly typical view being:

> They [the CPS] drop everything down a peg. The courts do this and the CPS know the courts are doing it and so they do the same. We are the only ones who get it right.

But even the officer quoted here conveyed his understanding of why the CPS tend to reduce the charge – and, implicitly, of why the CPS are better equipped than the police to assess the level of charge which can be sustained in court. For the most part, therefore, officers have re-defined their role so that the reality of CPS control over this stage of the prosecution process does not cause them great distress. It is just another among many limitations upon their own authority and freedom of action, to be viewed in the same light as, say, the requirement of obedience to a superior officer, or the fact that it is courts and not police officers who determine culpability and impose sentence. It is an inescapable element of their job and therefore not something to get annoyed at or to struggle against.

We would conclude, therefore, that, contrary to the impression conveyed by McConville *et al.* (1991: *passim*), the notion of police construction – while helpful in assisting us to come to terms with the reality of police investigation and case preparation – is liable seriously to mislead if we take it to mean that because the police are involved from the outset of the case[2] they effectively control the whole criminalisation process. From the police perspective their intimate acquaintanceship with the reality of criminal behaviour is constantly being overruled by higher authority. Police investigations are commonly frustrated; their judgements are commonly overruled. Nor is it true that the police devote all their energy to *incriminating* suspects. Certainly in respect of assault, the police construct innocence just as much as they construct guilt. Many of their constructions are *under*-constructions. The image of the police as effective manipulators of reality, building cases in such a way as to distort the truth, override suspect rights and incriminate the innocent needs to be set alongside the many difficulties and frustrations experienced by the police in dealing with staple criminal conduct such as assault, and their manifest *failure*, in the majority of cases, to marshal all the various actors in order to bring an inchoate event into that very special form of 'story' which will satisfy a court. This is a demanding exercise: it is a process which the police influence as best they can, but which they do not dominate and control.

Chapter 7

Victims in court

Trials are the showpiece of the criminal justice system and the focus of the trial is firmly upon the defendant. But in cases of assault successful prosecution depends almost invariably upon the victim. It is the victim, and very often the victim alone, who represents the substance of the prosecution case. It is true that the majority of convictions follow a guilty plea (McConville *et al.* 1991: 149), yet even in these cases the victim is of central importance: the defendant may plead guilty precisely because he or she perceives the complainant to be 'strong'; in other cases the prosecution may accept a plea to a lesser charge because they perceive the complainant to be 'weak'. And yet the victim's status is equivocal, apparently out of keeping with that person's importance to the prosecution case (Zedner 1994: 1232). In the event of a trial the victim's interests are often ignored (Walmsley 1986: 41). He or she has been described as a marginal, even a pariah-like figure (Rock 1993: 179). This is despite government rhetoric which proclaims the victim's interests to be at the heart of the justice system.[1] In this chapter we shall explore this conundrum. How is it possible for such scant consideration to be given to the victim's interests when he or she is so important to the prosecution case?

Since it was established in 1986 the Crown Prosecution Service has been responsible for all criminal prosecutions in England and Wales. The principal CPS criterion of success is conviction. The service must also, like any bureaucratic organisation, have an eye to the administrative value of efficient case management. The trial process is enormously costly; the rationing of trials is necessarily an important objective for the CPS. This means that it will not wish to pursue high-risk cases; second, it will wish to secure a high proportion of guilty pleas. The CPS criteria for determining whether to proceed with a prosecution are evidential sufficiency and the public interest. There is a problematic relationship between these criteria and the victim's own interest (as it may be) in having an assailant brought to trial. In fact the interests of the victim are held to be subsumed within the public interest.[2] The attitude of the victim is of course related to questions of evidential sufficiency. If a victim wishes to withdraw a complaint, or is ambivalent, his or her attitude has to be taken into account in considering whether or not there is likely to be evidence upon which to proceed. So decisions which appear to reflect responsiveness to the interests of the victim may in fact reflect the prosecutor's role as representative of a bureaucratic institution which must ration both its own and the court's resources. Like the police, the CPS will make judgements about the victim's reliability and ability to perform well in court. They will do this on the basis of information in the police file. This information may include not only 'hard' material, such as statements, photographs and medical evidence, but also 'soft' material such as an assessment of the victim's reliability.

According to McConville *et al.* (1991: 147), case review is marked by continued police dominance of decision-making:

> The CPS, far from being an independent agency, is a police-dependent body, confining review to evidence sufficiency questions, eschewing public interest criteria, utilizing the contradictory and malleable nature of the principles in the codes to further narrowly conceived objectives and, at its worst, adopting an uncritical support-the-police mandate.

Our research was conducted some four years after that of McConville and his colleagues and was confined to a study of assaults. Unlike them, we found the CPS influence to be pervasive, not least in determining the level of charge. To give one illustration of this, our sample included eleven initial s. 18 charges (GBH with intent). CPS reduction of an initial s. 18 charge appeared virtually standard. The eleven s. 18 charges produced just one conviction on that count.

Police officers whom we interviewed claimed that the CPS commonly reduced charges to a level which no longer reflects the true gravity of the assault. Our own case monitoring bore this out. We should emphasise that this is not of itself reason to criticise the CPS: the circumstances surrounding assaults can be difficult to penetrate, while victims' commitment to the prosecution cause cannot be relied on. Many cases therefore present evidential problems. In these circumstances it is tempting to reduce the level of charge in order to induce a guilty plea.

This may be done either at the stage of initial CPS case review or several weeks or months later, at court, as part of a plea bargain.[3] Of the twenty-nine cases in our sample which were prosecuted, nine (31 per cent) were the subject of an immediate guilty plea; nine (31 per cent) were the subject of a not guilty plea but the defendant pleaded in due course to a lesser charge; six (21 per cent) were aborted when the prosecution offered no evidence (or, in mid-trial, offered no *further* evidence); four defendants (14 per cent) were tried and found guilty; and one defendant (3 per cent) was acquitted. These figures indicate a substantial use of the plea-bargain.

The question then arises: whose interests are served by the plea-bargain? The answer is not altogether clear. Take, for example, the case of Patrick Dashwood (3). Four suspects were charged with both assault and public order offences. The case was listed for trial at the Crown Court where, on the day of the trial, a bargain was struck: all charges were dropped against one defendant and the others pleaded to violent disorder. It is possible to analyse this and many other cases from a variety of perspectives. Taking first the defendants, the decision to allow one defendant to walk free (arguably, he was the prime mover in the whole affair) and to proceed against the other three smacked of expediency at best. The convicted men were indignant at this: they regarded their co-defendant as someone whom they had gone to help and who had then turned his back on them. From their point of view therefore justice was not served. The investigating officer, on the other hand, was more than content with the plea-bargain. He did not mind that the assault charges were dropped, because violent disorder is a serious charge in itself. He also did not mind that the charges against one defendant were dropped entirely. This was because he considered the case against him to have been weak. All in all he regarded three out of four as a good 'result'. The barristers, both prosecuting and defending, and the judge were likewise well satisfied. All were pleased at not having to conduct the trial.

If, however, we consider the *public* interest, there is reason to be less sanguine. Taking first the need to ensure efficient case management, the fact that the plea-bargain was secured only on the morning of the trial meant that considerable public expenditure had already been incurred, even if aborting the trial did assist the administration of the court: indeed, the fact that each of these defendants had his own barrister highlighted the waste of resources endemic in the court process. Second, in respect of the denunciatory or symbolic purpose of criminal justice, there was no public examination of this very violent event. As in so many other cases, justice was done in corridors. And what of the victims? As far as they were concerned the late plea-bargain brought only belated relief. They had experienced the burden of anticipating the trial over the preceding 12 months, their anxiety relieved only at the eleventh hour after they had endured a whole morning in the court waiting area, subject to verbal threats and menacing gestures from friends of their assailants. Nor had they been party to the negotiations leading to the plea-bargain. They were present, but not consulted. For the victims, therefore, the court experience constituted both a relief and a disappointment.

The Royal Commission on Criminal Justice recorded some disagreement among lawyers concerning the victim's role and was divided on the question of the proper degree of contact between victims and prosecuting counsel.[4] While it recommended that the CPS respond to the victim's need for information about the case (RCCJ, 8.40), direct contact between CPS prosecutors (or barristers acting on their behalf) and victims was regarded as problematic (RCCJ, 8.41). The prevailing view is that there must be no question of partisanship as far as the prosecution is concerned (Rock 1993: 170), a doctrine which may, as Rock has shown, have unfortunate consequences for the victim in court. It is to be expected therefore that victims will remain in ignorance of decisions relating to charges and to the acceptance of pleas; these will be presented as *faits accomplis* with no acknowledgement that the victim has a legitimate interest in what is going on.

While victims may be affronted by their marginalisation in court, our research suggests that the technicalities of the law (represented, for instance, in the distinctions between s. 18, s. 20 and s. 47 charges) have little or no meaning as far as most victims are concerned. Being only too well aware of the 'otherness' of the law as expressed in its rules, culture and language they are content to let the police and the courts decide these matters. But while victims may be happy to accept that the initial charge is the right one – they are unlikely to have any basis for deciding otherwise – they are much less likely to accept the legitimacy of the decision to *reduce* the charge (Shapland *et al.* 1985: 79). A reduction in the charge gives the assault victim the message that prosecutor and court have downgraded the level of harm he or she has experienced. Considerations which carry weight with the CPS (as for instance that the new charge will permit a sentence similar to that which would have been imposed had the charge remained at its original level[5]) may not impress the victim. The Director of Victim Support has stated that

Victim Support receives frequent complaints that victims who have suffered a serious offence are distressed when the offender is convicted on a lesser charge to which he has pleaded. Many victims would prefer the seriousness of the offence against them to be recognised by a plea of guilty to the full charge.[6]

This is consistent with the findings of our research. It reflects the fact that victims are seeking *vindication*. They will not feel vindicated if the defendant pleads to a lesser charge and is then 'let off' with what they consider a derisory sentence. Courts are all about symbolism, but the actual symbolic content is not necessarily that which is intended. Courts cannot avoid delivering vindication and humiliation, but they can determine *who* is vindicated and who is humiliated: it appears to some victims that they are treated as of no account while their assailant is accorded a minor triumph.

As we have already indicated, the practice of reducing charges may be defended on the basis that the defendant can still be sentenced 'for what he's done'. We ourselves observed cases which appeared to support the thesis that courts sentence on the 'story' rather than the charge. That is to say, they imposed stiff sentences upon defendants whose charges had been plea-bargained down. For example, Melotti (69) had originally faced four charges – two of ABH and two of GBH. Before the case was heard the prosecuting barrister explained to us that he was prepared to drop the GBH charges down a notch because there was a 'strong' judge on the bench who would ensure that Melotti 'would still get a proper sentence . . . he'll be sentenced for what he's done'. The barrister pointed out that the ABH charge permitted a maximum sentence of five years' imprisonment – the same as for a s. 20 charge. So he clearly believed that, at least before certain judges, assailants would be sentenced on the prosecution 'story' rather than on the charge. This is what seems to have happened in this case. Melotti was dealt with much more severely than other defendants who, at least in our eyes, had inflicted greater harm. It did indeed appear that the reduced charge had not secured a better outcome for the defendant. Another case from which we might draw this conclusion was that of the assault on Rowena Macintosh (66). The ABH charges in this case were plea-bargained down to common assault. But the defendant was fined £150 on each count and ordered to pay compensation to each of his victims. This again was a more severe penalty than was suffered by other defendants who were convicted on a s. 47 or even a s. 20 count. So again one might question whether the defendant benefited from the plea-bargain which had been struck. If it is generally true that defendants are sentenced on the story rather than the charge, one might conclude that they would be better advised to take their chances at trial rather than accede to a plea-bargain.

In fact our evidence on this point is equivocal. Some cases support the 'sentencing on the story rather than the charge' hypothesis, while others do not. Perhaps the most powerful contra-indication was the assault on the policeman, Ronald Pratt (28). This was a serious assault and the initial charge of s. 20 GBH seemed appropriate. But on the morning of the trial we discovered that the assailant, Daniel Howard, faced only a charge of ABH. Even Howard's solicitor was surprised at this. He had seen the photographs of the victim and he told us, without equivocation: "It's GBH." One may speculate as to why the CPS was prepared to offer what appeared to us a generous plea-bargain. Perhaps it was in the belief that Howard too would be sentenced on the story rather than the charge – and of course it is true that the court has ample sentencing powers even in respect of s. 47. But in this instance the reduction in the charge gave the judge a loophole which he proved keen to exploit. Howard was given a suspended prison sentence. It is doubtful whether the judge, although disposed to be lenient, would have felt able to impose a non-custodial sentence in respect of GBH upon a police officer, particularly given that Howard was an habitual violent offender.

So we appear to have a very mixed picture. Where there is a gap between story and charge – either a severe charge and a low-key story, or a modest charge and an unpleasant story – the sentence imposed will sometimes reflect the story and sometimes it will reflect the charge. This is hardly surprising: sentencing is not consistent in any event. The outcomes of our own small sample of convicted assaults is given in Table 7.1. It can be seen that there is *some* relationship between charge and sentence, but the overall impression is that the level of charge is a very *weak* predictor of the sentence that the court will impose.

It could be argued that the distinction between s. 47 and s. 20 reflects the injuries sustained rather than the question of intent, in which case it might be appropriate that the assailant be sentenced on 'the story' since the degree of culpability is not necessarily reflected in the charge. But what if the CPS decision to substitute a lower charge – perhaps in the course of a plea-bargain – influences 'the story' of the assault as this is presented in court? The cost of the plea-bargain to the justice process might in that case be significant – and no longer defensible. Unsurprisingly, few CPS lawyers or prosecuting barristers would accept that 'stories' are doctored to fit a reduced charge. But police officers claimed that this happened on occasion, and our own observations bore them out.

Table 7.1 Eventual outcome matched against charge upon which conviction based

	s. 18 GBH	s. 20 GBH	s. 47 ABH
Conditional discharge	–	–	2(22%)
Probation/Community Service	–	4(50%)	2(22%)
Fine	–	3(37.5%)	2(22%)
Suspended prison sentence	–	–	2(22%)
Prison	1(100%)	1(12.5%)	1(11%)
Total	1	8	9

One example was the prosecution of Anthony Niblett's assailant (33). Here the initial charge was one of GBH, but this was plea-bargained down to ABH to which the assailant, Mather, pleaded guilty. The plea-bargain having been concluded, there was no attempt to convey to the court the true severity of Niblett's injuries. These were said to comprise a hairline fracture to the cheekbone, temporary loss of consciousness, and a cut cheek. In fact Niblett had been hospitalised and had missed several weeks' work. It seemed to us that the reduced charge inhibited the prosecution from giving a full account of the injuries suffered by Niblett, and this in turn enabled the defence to present the incident as a fight in which one of the two men had happened to come off worst. This was reflected in the magistrates' approach to sentencing Mather, when the minor motoring offences for which he was dealt with at the same time were given greater prominence in the chairman's peroration. They also attracted a larger fine.

The suggestion that 'the story' is tailored to a reduced charge is bound to be contentious, and it is difficult to demonstrate empirically. But we would contend that it is almost inevitable that where a charge is reduced below a level merited by the victim's actual injury (as happened in several of the cases which we followed) the prosecution will be inclined to downplay the incident. *Not* to do this would convey a very confusing message to the court – why, if the violence was greater than suggested by the revised charge, did the prosecution consent to the plea-bargain? We would conclude, therefore, that the 'guilty plea system', as it has been styled, does not only affect charge and sentence – it may also contribute to a distorted account of the offending behaviour.

DIFFICULTIES FACED BY THE PROSECUTION IN PROVING ASSAULT CHARGES

It is generally assumed that the courts could not possibly process the present volume of cases (or anything approaching it) were not the great majority of defendants to plead guilty. 'Settlement' of one form or another is a feature of all branches of the court system and many would argue that it is the legal system's most dominant characteristic. But another encouragement to settlement – that is to say, to plea-bargaining – is that trials involve risk. Most defendants plead guilty, but of those who do not some 17 per cent are acquitted.[7] The burden of proof in any trial lies with the prosecution. The task of the defence is to cast doubt on the prosecution case, perhaps supplying a rival account (Rock 1993: 33). The defence case does not have to be as 'solid' as that of the prosecution. Merely by undermining the impression conveyed by the prosecution and the prosecution witnesses, defence counsel may persuade the jury that they cannot be sure of the truth of the prosecution case. According to Rock, 'in the relatively sealed world of the court room, where stories and their tellers were all there was to judge, doubt did not seem very difficult to introduce' (*ibid.*: 34).

This was our impression also. What is more, it seemed to us that assaults, with their susceptibility to the presentation of a rival, completely contradictory account, had their own specially problematic features. Even in what appeared to the investi- gating police officer (and perhaps to us) an 'open and shut' case, the defence might still succeed in casting doubt. Take, for example, the trial of Roy Camp (20), who faced alternative counts of s. 18 and s. 20 assault upon publican Timothy Cooper. This was a close run thing despite the prosecution having produced an impressive witness in support of Cooper's own unshakeable account.

In part this was because although Cooper remembered the 'glassing', his recollection of events in the pub leading up to his confrontation with Camp was less sure. He contradicted himself a number of times, albeit in respect of peripheral matters. Also, his oral evidence departed in some minor particulars from his written statement. The defence seized on this, lengthy cross-examination being devoted to the period preceding the assault. By concentrating upon these minor inconsistencies and focusing minutely upon matters of detail, the defence succeeded, so it seemed to us, in creating an aura of doubt around Cooper's evidence. There could be little doubt that Camp had in fact injured Cooper: the circumstantial evidence was strong – both Cooper and the other prosecution witness gave clear, unshakeable accounts of the actual assault; and yet an element of doubt was introduced, both in our minds and in the minds of the jury, who deliberated for some hours. The fact that this can happen where the evidence is so strong gives some indication of the difficulties faced by the prosecution in pursuing more problematic cases in which, for example, the complainant or other witnesses are of damaged status – in having, for example, a criminal record of their own or perhaps in having been assaulted in dubious circumstances.

Certain categories of assault are more difficult to prove than others. The breakdown in respect of the assault archetypes which we identified is given in Table 7.2. From this it can be seen that robberies and other street attacks, 'domestic' assaults, and assaults committed by drugs dealers are *least* likely to lead to conviction, whereas assaults following a dispute (say between motorists) or assaults which are committed against people 'in role' (police officers, ambulancemen, publicans) are most likely to be prosecuted effectively. The success of the last two categories reflects victim commitment and the comparatively low cost to the victim of co-operating with the prosecuting authorities. There is also, in the case of role-based attacks, the determination of the police to protect those classes of victim who may be considered vulnerable because of the nature of their employment, or with whom the police have some affinity (not least, their fellow officers). The low conviction rate for robberies and street attacks reflects the low detection rate. As far as 'domestic' violence and violence in the drugs world are concerned, the low conviction rate is a direct result of victims' inability or unwilling-ness to make a formal complaint or to give evidence when called upon to do so. In other words, this high failure rate is not necessarily reflected in the trial: most cases do not get that far. Nonetheless, where there *is* a trial the intrinsic vulnerability of the prosecution case may be starkly revealed. Victims and other witnesses who have been carefully nurtured by the police and the CPS up to that point may conclude that the dubious benefits of testifying against their assailant are outweighed by the all too evident costs. Prosecutors have plenty of experience of this: it is some-thing which they bear in mind as they contemplate inviting a plea to a lesser charge.

Because our own research was focused on victims rather than upon defendants it was inevitable that we were more attuned to obstacles to proving an assault charge, and to prosecution shortcomings in over-coming those obstacles, than we were to weaknesses in the conduct of the defence case. This is a bias arising from our research method, and one that is difficult to avoid: *all* social research findings are influenced

Table 7.2 Outcome by case category

	Robbery/ street attacks	History of hostile acquaintanceship	Arising from dispute	Pub/club violence	Drugs world	Sexual partner or other 'domestic'	Role-based attacks
No police contact	4(14%)	–	1(12.5%)	7(37%)	–	6(31.5%)	3(43%)
No 'complaint' or complaint not sustained	10(36%)	2(28.5%)	2(25%)	6(31.5%)	3(100%)	8(42%)	–
Case not detected or not proceeded with by police	10(38%)	1(14%)	2(25%)	1(5%)	–	–	–
Case dropped by CPS	–	2(28.5%)	–	–	–	1(5%)	–
Not guilty	–	–	–	–	–	1(5%)	–
Successful prosecution	4(14%)	2(28.5%)	3(37.5%)	5(26%)	–	3(15%)	4(57%)
Total	28	7	8	19	3	19	7

by the researchers' choice of informants. In our case this means that we have barely addressed the criticism of defence lawyers (made, for example, by McConville *et al.* 1991: 167) to the effect that they are 'part of, rather than challengers to, the apparatus of criminal justice', thereby failing to protect their clients against the crime control values of the justice system. That is not to say that we think that this perspective has no validity, or is not worthy of development. It is just that we ourselves are not well placed to develop it. But one might say that there is implied corroboration of this thesis in the fact that, *although proving assault is difficult*, there is nonetheless a high conviction rate overall. Twenty-two convictions from ninety-three cases, as in our sample, is indeed an impressive 'strike rate' when compared with conviction rates in respect of, say, burglary, car theft, or sexual assault. This of course reflects the fact that a high proportion of assailants are identifiable by their victims or by other witnesses. In fact we observed convictions in respect of what appeared to us to be weak cases, although, just as one might expect, these were secured on the defendant's guilty plea rather than following a trial. In the cases of David Thompson (71) and Michael Tapper (19) the defendants pleaded guilty to GBH when they might well have hoped for the substitution of a lesser charge. The investigating officer in Tapper's case commented:

> If I was a solicitor I'd tell him to plead guilty to an ABH and not guilty to a GBH and if the prosecutor . . . was not happy with that I would elect trial by jury. Almost certainly it'd be reduced to ABH at Crown Court and he'd probably walk away with a bind-over.

But Tapper's assailant, who pleaded guilty before the magistrates, apparently opted for a speedy resolution. Thompson's attacker likewise pleaded guilty to charges which were admitted by the investigating officer to be 'on the high side'. A third example occurred in the case of the three men accused of assaulting Patrick Dashwood and his friends (3): one of the defendants, Daniels, pleaded guilty to volent disorder despite the fact that the evidence against him was not strong (and included a legally controversial 'dock identification'). The officer in the case had not expected Daniels to be convicted given the weak identification evidence against him. One might well conclude that the defendant was ill-served by his solicitor and barrister.

THE 'STORY' AND THE COURT

Rock (1993: 31) has described the manner in which trials involve the deployment of a public language and a paring down of both the defendant's and the victim's behaviour in order to formulate the few pivotal allegations that comprise the case. Whether or not the defendant is found guilty (and perhaps even where he or she enters a guilty plea), doubts may remain as to context, motivation, and even the extent of the harm. 'The facts at issue' are likely to be a deliberate simplification, obscuring some issues and illuminating others. The presentation of the case tends to strip away context and history. It ignores 'many of the tangled social relations, hurts, incidents, motives and emotions that could be woven into personal disputes, concentrating on but a few' (*ibid.*: 31). Rock observes of the trial that it is intended to 'shed greyness and ambiguity . . . amplifying the differences between protagonists, focusing on the circumstantial and the situational, and offering a stark argument for fault-finding and judgment' (*ibid.*: 32). Prosecution and defence accounts have to be unambiguous, one-dimensional and static – in other words, not reflecting the experience of participants and observers.

This trimming of events to fit the court process is manifest also in the snapshot quality of criminal justice. In preparing what Rock refers to as 'an object for the court' the history and complexity of an event is lost. This is especially a feature of those cases in which there is a history of violence – archetypally, the 'domestic' case. Unless the defendant is charged with more than one offence it is difficult for the prosecution to convey to the court the history of a violent relationship. An assault by a man upon his partner or former partner will be presented as an isolated incident. The court is unlikely to be given any insight into the causes of the violence, the motivations of the participants, or the balance of culpability. By excluding material which is, according to the conventions of the court, irrelevant, the trial in turn becomes 'irrelevant' to the victim.

This has costs in terms of fairness and, second, in limiting the dramatic and, one might say, the therapeutic potential of the court process. Fairness, in the sense of doing justice to the accounts of both victim and defendant, is an inevitable casualty of the guilty plea system. The potential costs to the defendant are well documented (Baldwin and McConville 1977: *passim*) and we have made brief reference to them. The costs to the victim are less commented upon, but certainly in respect of assault, guilty pleas can permit a distorted account of the violence and of its background in terms of the parties' relationship. To return to the assault upon Anthony Niblett, when the defendant pleaded guilty to a s. 47 charge (reduced from s. 20) the prosecution failed to challenge the defence claim that Niblett had struck the first blow, although this was something which Niblett vehemently denied. Following this, the defence solicitor was able to argue that his client had merely over-reacted to Niblett's provocative behaviour. This was one among several cases in which highly contentious accounts of behaviour and motivation were allowed to stand.[8] Where the defendant pleads guilty the victim is seldom in court to hear the defence plea in mitigation. That is perhaps just as well, although some victims *are* present and are affronted by what they hear. There is also the possibility that the unchallenged defence account will be reported in the press.[9]

The failure of the criminal process to achieve its dramatic or therapeutic potential is less commented upon, but arguably it is of greater significance since it encompasses all criminal proceedings, including trials. It is well known that trials are in general a lot less exciting than they appear on television (Bottoms and McClean 1976: 226; Christie 1986a). Christie has specifically attacked the failure of the criminal process to achieve its dramatic potential, arguing that the drama of the courtroom does not reflect basic values, or expose conflicts, or create doubt. Instead, it over-simplifies; it is avowedly utilitarian; and it attempts to convey clear, simple-minded messages. Our own observations are consistent with this: we were especially struck by the banality of proceedings in the magistrates' courts. Cases dealt with in these courts are typically attended by muddle and procedural confusion. The business of sentencing an offender found guilty on a number of counts may be done in such a way as to make it impossible to determine which sentence relates to which charge. Motoring offences become muddled up with assaults. The potential impact upon an assailant of being confronted with the harm which he or she has done to another person is lost in the bathos of administrative detail. In these circumstances one can only be relieved if the victim is not present.

Even where there is a trial it may be difficult for anyone other than the lawyers to feel engaged in the process. The main reason for this, certainly in respect of assault, is the tendency to translate moral issues into technical legal argument. The trial of Michael Addis (2) was a striking instance of this disjunction between the originating drama and the focus of the trial, the latter hinging upon the definition of 'intent' and 'recklessness'. These semantic questions had little relevance for the victim, Matthew Saunders, and they clearly perplexed the jury. Saunders had lost the sight of one eye in the course of the attack and he had also, before that, lost his girlfriend of 15 years to his assailant. There were issues of immense importance to Saunders which needed at some point to be addressed. These included: the scope for financial compensation; the resolution of his rupture with his girlfriend and of his relationship with Addis; and his need for some public acknowledgement that he had suffered a grievous wrong. He may also have wished to see Addis punished. The trial failed to do any of these things and, through the narrowness of its focus, culminated in a 'not guilty' verdict which evidently caused the jury some unease – principally, we would surmise, because it failed to give public acknowledgement to the harm suffered by the victim. In this case the options offered to the jury were such that they felt unable to find Addis guilty as charged despite their awareness that he had inflicted terrible injury on Saunders. They had a choice to make between different constructions of the incident, with no possibility of their verdict reflecting the competing perceptions and the complexity of real life.

The trial is bound, as Christie suggests, to over-simplify in that it is not designed primarily to discover 'what happened' in any sense that a lay person might understand. Its purpose is rather to test the defendant's guilt in relation to a specific charge. This process is intended to achieve certainty in respect of narrowly defined issues, but trials tend to leave a residue of doubt (Pannick 1987: 53). As far as the defence is concerned, that is often their function. The defence lawyer demands a more or less coherent exculpatory story from his client, a story which should have some prospect of public credibility. The trial pits one story against another. Dramatic interest is sustained through anticipation of the jury's verdict, but this is an kind of artificial tension generated by the legal process itself. Other than that, court proceedings tend to alienate. The procedures of the court are distant from the parties' own world, which means that they have an arbitrary relationship to the originating event. In itself the trial is an intense and probably an unpleasant experience, but it takes place in a vacuum, removed from the dramatic and painful incident of which it is supposed to be the culmination and resolution. This supports the defendant in his or her self-absorption, while the victim discovers that the court deals with his or her 'story' only in a tangential way. The trial is an artefact. It addresses the court's concerns, not those of the victim.

THE VICTIM IN COURT

The victim/witness is likely to spend most of his or her time at court not actually in the courtroom but in corridors or waiting rooms. There that person will experience the delays and frustrations which make even a court officer's day burdensome. Courts are places where everybody spends a good deal of time waiting for something to happen (Rock 1993: 277). The victim/witness will spend this time in a public place, possibly with no access to food or drink, and in proximity to the defendant and his or her supporters.[10] If the victim/witness is lucky he or she may be accompanied by a guardian police officer, but the protection afforded by the police is variable: the 'big' cases generate a fairly effective police cordon, but most assault victims will have no one assigned to them. If they do have a police officer in attendance, circumstances dictate that conversation with the officer is likely to be sparse. The victim may be kept in ignorance of how long he or she will have to wait, or what the delay signifies. It is then not uncommon, having perhaps waited all day, for the victim to find that the case has been adjourned. Having steeled him- or herself to give evidence the victim will then be required to screw his or her courage to the sticking point once again. This is trying even for those with great respect for the law and its processes. Where a victim is more ambivalent in attitude, or where the victim's lifestyle is not well-ordered, he or she may find the court's demands unsustainable.

A peculiar feature of victims' experience at court is that they are granted no special status by professional court users. Having come to court in furtherance of 'their' case they will find that their own stake in the proceedings is barely acknowledged. They are just witnesses – and witnesses, although vital to the success of the prosecution case, are firmly excluded from the intimacies of the professionals' world. Rock has described the marginalisation of the victim in court (1993: 179), as has Shapland (1983) who refers to the victim as a 'non-person'. Rock argues that victims are perceived by the professionals to have an 'almost baneful' influence. They are in the awkward position of being essential to the success of the prosecution case but also a threat to it in that there is always a risk that their evidence might be contaminated through conversation with other witnesses or with the police or prosecutor. Accordingly, victims had to be:

> kept somewhat at bay. Together with others collectively labelled 'the public' . . . they were thrust to a distance, never fully trusted, denied knowledge about much of what transpired, relegated to the safe, outer margins of the court's social organization.
>
> (*Ibid.*: 179)

Given this experience, the victim is bound to conclude that any vestige of ownership of the case has finally been removed.

It is not only in the waiting area that the victim/witness may feel threatened by the defendant and his or her supporters. Defendants, especially if they are jointly charged and stand together in the dock, can dominate a courtroom by their deportment. Displays of dumb insolence and gestures to supporters on the spectators' benches, perhaps noisily reciprocated, can establish an air of menace only barely kept in check. This is especially true in the magistrates' courts. The formality of the proceedings is less marked; the spectators are closer to the body of the court. Profiting from this, defendants such as those in the cases of Dashwood (3) and Freeman (4) appeared relaxed, defiant and unimpressed by the majesty of the law. This was achieved without any flagrant challenge to the authority of the court.

The ability of defendants to dominate, perhaps with the assistance of partisan spectators, is assisted by the geography of the courtroom. The defendant in the dock, flanked by police officers (and sometimes accompanied by fellow-defendants) is comparatively protected, whereas the witness can appear solitary and exposed. Rock refers to the lonely prominence of the witness box, in which the witness is in full view of the jury, the defendant and the spectators. According to Rock, prosecution witnesses frequently claimed that defendants silently menaced them as they testified (*ibid.*: 50). The influence of spectators is perhaps more apparent to the independent observer because spectators are typically less restrained in their behaviour than is the defendant in the dock. Spectators at a trial may belong to either camp or to none, but in several of the trials which we observed the public gallery was heavily colonised by supporters of the defendant with the result that the victim had to run the gauntlet of hostile gestures and *sotto voce* remarks.

Cross-examination

The most dramatic form of exposure undergone by the victim is the experience of cross-examination. This is the point at which the victim's equivocal status as *alleged* victim is most obviously underlined. The defence barrister's questions may be construed as an attack upon his or her character and lifestyle, at least as much as a challenge to the substance of his or her evidence. As Rock points out, the process of giving evidence and of cross-examination does not serve to vindicate the witness's alleged wrongs, nor is it intended to do so. Rather it is intended to test the charges on the indictment. So victims, once transformed into witnesses for the prosecution, may themselves become defensive, indignant and confused. They may feel frightened and alone, unsure of what is happening to them and in need of reassurance, both practical and symbolic. Shapland (1984) claimed that while victims experience many unpleasantnesses in court, they do not appear to find the experience of giving evidence to be a cause of great distress. Our own observations, and those of Paul Rock, invite a contrary view – at least in respect of the *assault* victim.

As the prime witness and therefore the pivot of the prosecution case the victim is almost inevitably challenged by the defence concerning his or her veracity, disinterestedness, integrity, knowledgeability, way of life, reputation and associations (Rock, 1993: 34). The judge will seldom intervene when a witness becomes distressed.[11] Judges do not see it as part of their duty to defend witnesses against telling questions which could be vital to the defendant's case. As a result, and as a matter of course, gravely wounding allegations may be put to witnesses in the most ordinary trial.

Rock's observations, and our own, contrast starkly with some of the advice given to victims in anticipation of a trial. For example, the Avon and Somerset Constabulary booklet issued to domestic assault victims says at one point: 'Remember a court is just a place where you explain what happened. You are not on trial.' While factually correct, this statement nonetheless gives a misleading impression of the victim's actual experience. Take the case of David Freeman (4). At the committal proceedings the *prosecution* barrister – not the defence – began in startling fashion: 'Ma'am, David Freeman is a bad man who, on his own admission, has been supplying drugs.' This set the tone, both for the committal and for the eventual trial. Freeman's cross-examination focused entirely upon his involvement in the drugs world. As an observer one almost forgot the assault which he had suffered. The effect of the cross-examination was to reinforce the impression that Freeman was thoroughly embedded in the criminal world of drug dealing so that his assault and abduction – if they had happened at all – were the acts of one set of criminals upon another. Freeman was trying to implicate others, but he was at least as guilty as they. In fact the effect of the cross-examination was to present Freeman as a 'grass' rather than as an assault victim. Throughout the proceedings it felt as if Freeman himself was on trial. In fact he was on trial twice over: he was being condemned by the 'straight' world of the courtroom *and* by the criminal underworld which he was trying to escape. This was evident from Freeman's demeanour. His whole manner indicated that he was being humiliated.

The defence managed to demonstrate again and again that Freeman was quite capable of lying – indeed, was an habitual liar. Freeman had considerable difficulty in remaining calm in the face of this sustained attack, lasting 50 minutes or so. He became progressively more sulky and his answers became ever shorter. By the end of the cross-examination one was bound to conclude that Freeman's credibility had been damaged, if only because he had appeared evasive in the witness box. It would not be surprising had the jury come to regard him with scepticism. To us it seemed that this was not because of anything in Freeman's past which had been revealed to the jury, but rather because of the way in which he had behaved before their very eyes. The object of the attack on Freeman may not have been to disprove the specific points of his story but rather to get him to act in this petulant fashion. It was to be expected that the defence barristers would prove more skilled at this kind of impression management than was Freeman himself.

In the course of the same trial we observed one of the basic techniques of cross-examination – a technique which can cause much anxiety to witnesses. This involves the practice of confronting the witness with discrepancies between his or her account newly given in court and the original statement to the police. By playing on the discrepancies between these two accounts the defence has an excellent opportunity to inject doubt into the prosecution case (Rock 1993: 44). In Freeman's case his evidence was supported by that of one other member of the drugs underworld, Michael Harrison. Harrison had at one point alleged that five members of the drugs gang who assaulted Freeman had entered the squat in which he had been 'dealing'. Then he said the number was four, and then at other times he seemed to refer to only three (the three who were on trial). Harrison eventually confirmed that four members of the gang had been present. The barrister hammered away at this inconsistency. He treated it as if Harrison could not remember whether he had invited six or eight friends to a dinner party – a truly incredible lapse of memory. He invited the jury to be dumbfounded that Harrison should forget the number of gang members who had arrived at the squat 12 months ago. To us this did not seem so incredible, but it was nonetheless possible that the aggressive questioning to which Harrison was subjected had shaken his evidence. The barrister had ascribed a certainty and exactitude to the witness's signed statement which any experienced observer would have known it could not possibly carry. He built his case around minor inconsistencies and in doing this he attempted to cast doubt on the witness's integrity. To us this felt like a clash of cultures – between the narrowly legalistic stance adopted by the defence barristers and the rather muddled account of a 12-month-old assault as remembered through a haze of heroin and cocaine addiction – which is what we were offered by Harrison and Freeman.

The background to this assault, and in particular the violence which Freeman's assailants were habitually prepared to employ, meant that Freeman's resolve was tested to the utmost. The demands made upon him were then compounded by the inefficiencies of court listing as the judge found that he could not complete the trial because he was scheduled to go on holiday. He therefore ordered a re-trial. Having given evidence at committal and at trial Freeman was expected to go into the witness box a third time. We were not surprised when both he and Harrison failed to put in an appearance at the second trial, forcing the prosecution to offer no evidence against the three defendants. It was difficult to imagine a worse outcome: even the most cynical plea-bargain would have been preferable. Certainly Freeman derived nothing but humiliation from the whole affair. Observation of this and other trials of non-stranger assault led us to the broad conclusion that victims' reluctance to stay the prosecution course is not, in terms of their own personal interests, misguided.

The victim and the sentence

The Royal Commission acknowledged the need to ensure victims' 'free cooperation' with the prosecution process (8.36). Accordingly it made broadly non-controversial recommendations concerning support for victims in court;[12] wider implementation of s. 23 of the Criminal Justice Act 1988 under which written evidence may be accepted where a witness is in justified fear of giving oral evidence; the speeding up of sensitive cases; and provision of more information to victims in the period prior to the court hearing. The Commission also recommended the creation of a new offence of witness intimidation in an attempt to tackle a problem regularly reported in the media.[13] If implemented, these provisions might do something to improve the lot of assault victims called upon to give evidence in a criminal trial. What the Commission did not do, and would doubtless have considered beyond its remit, was to consider how far crime victims might have a legitimate interest in decisions relating to the trial and punishment of someone whose alleged offence, they are bound to feel, was committed against *them* rather than against 'the state'. It is not our purpose here to consider arguments for and against victim involvement in the sentencing process,[14] except to say that we see no case for the victim's views being determinative but a very strong case for the victim's experience of the crime and its aftermath being conveyed directly to the court.[15] This applies particularly to victims of violence since the prosecution of assault relies so heavily upon the victim's commitment to the process, often at considerable personal cost. To argue in these circumstances that the victim's experience and views are irrelevant to the court's deliberations is quixotic – either that or it betrays a lack of understanding concerning the central role of the victim in determining whether or not an assault should be prosecuted.

Arguments that the victim should be granted a stronger voice are consistent with the views of such as Nils Christie, who laments the disappearance of the victim and the appropriation of the 'conflict' by agents of the state (Christie 1977). One means by which the victim may be granted a voice in court is through the provision of 'victim impact statements', now introduced at the sentencing stage in many states in the USA. Fifteen US states also permit the victim to remain in court after giving evidence, while four allow this throughout the proceedings (Kelly 1990). Despite these innovations, Kelly observes that few victims receive any benefit from them. Less than 3 per cent of victims exercise their right to attend court proceedings or to make 'impact' or opinion statements. She concludes that the reforms have merely tinkered with the problem of victim disempowerment, being for the most part 'well-kept secrets that few victims know about or use to their advantage' (*ibid.*).

In the UK the idea of victim impact statements has encountered strong resistance from within the legal establishment and from academic commentators (Ashworth 1993: 27). Brief consideration was given to the topic in the *Victim's Charter*, where it was dismissed in a fusillade of scepticism:

> Is this a good idea in principle? How would it be put into effect? Would reports be given in every case, or only when the victim asks for one? Who would make them?

The fundamental objection to victim impact statements rests on a view of victims as introducing an *erratic* element into the trial process, with victims being seen as the embodiment of private vengeance – this being what the 'offence against society' model is designed to overcome. The state punishes offenders in order that justice may be consistently applied and vengeance eliminated. All the various theories of justice, whether utilitarian or retributive, express the state's interest. Victim participation is associated with emotionality, and hence with *in*justice.

One way in which the justice system *has* sought to respond to the needs of crime victims is through ordering the offender to pay financial compensation. This is an apparent departure from the 'offence against society' model, but has been defended as contributing both to the *reintegration* of the offender and to the restoration of the victim's *dominion* (Braithwaite and Pettit 1990: 91). Courts now have a statutory duty to explain their failure to make a compensation order.[16] They are also required to give priority to compensation over a fine.[17] But in practice the victim has such a low profile in court that the prosecutor may make no reference to compensation (Hough 1991) even when the offender has the means to pay. Of the twenty cases in our sample in which the defendant was sentenced specifically for *assault*, a compensation order was made in ten. The amount required to be paid was unpredictable, even random: calculations as to the defendant's ability to pay were based on evidence which was both frail and incomplete. Some awards were swingeing (£2,000 for the broken jaw suffered by Edward Jones (25)), while others appeared little more than token. Compensation awards are such a marginal feature of the sentencing process that few assault victims had given the possibility much thought. It certainly was not a priority, even where there was a strong sense that the assailant should be brought to account. None of the victims whose cases we followed had supported a prosecution in the hope of restitution, although that is not to say that they would not have welcomed reimbursement of the costs incurred as a result of the attack, say for dental treatment or for loss of earnings. But most assault victims have modest expectations of their assailant – or of the court – in this regard.

What is it, then, that assault victims want from the court? Much has been made of the finding that crime victims are not, in general, especially punitive (Shapland *et al.* 1985; Hough and Moxon 1985).[18] On the basis of our own research we would say something rather different. Most of the victims whom we interviewed *had no ideas at all* about the sentence which should be imposed on their assailant, always supposing that he or she be brought before the court. Most were aware of the principal sentencing options and, if pushed, would plump for one or other of these, but it generally appeared that their heart was not in it. We would suggest that this is because the sentencing options currently available lack resonance as far as assault victims are concerned. They have heard of prisons, fines, and probation – perhaps even of community service – but they tend not to think in these terms themselves. These sentencing options, although known, appear distant and psychologically unsatisfying. Victims know what they are, but they find it difficult to relate them to their own experience. Of course it might be argued that this does not matter: sentencing is the public exercise of authority by the state. Sentences are not meant to resonate with victims; they are meant to serve retributive or utilitarian purposes. Nonetheless it tends to be assumed that the punishments meted out in court make sense to victims. On the whole we do not believe they do. Many of the assault victims whom we interviewed had no discernible views as to what should happen in court; but for a victim to have 'no views' in response to being knocked senseless is inconceivable. This illustrates the degree to which the justice process is insulated from normal, everyday notions about what is fair or reasonable. The 'event' then becomes the property of professionals; the victims have no further role and, because they are afforded no role – and are trained to *accept* that they have no role – they have no views. As far as the justice of their case is concerned, they have suffered a lobotomy. It is comparable to the Income Support claimant who has no views on Social Security policy: it is a failure of the sociological imagination, an inability to relate the private trouble to the public issue (Mills 1959: 10). Since most people are not sociologists the fact that the criminalisation of assault is handled in a way which makes no sense to them personally goes unchallenged.

At the same time we would not posit an absolute division between private and public interests within the justice process. Our contact with assault victims revealed that the denunciatory function of punishment has meaning for many. They also talk in terms of wanting their assailant to understand what it is that he has done to them. So it is possible for some element of remedy for the private wrong to be contained within the public response. If greater emphasis were to be placed upon these aspects of the criminal process the 'offence against society' model would meet the needs of at least some victims. This tends not to happen at the moment because sentencing is so much a utilitarian exercise – with the emphasis upon public rather than private utility. There is of course a connection between the sentencing process and victim purposes such as public denunciation of the offender and getting him or her to understand the harm that has been done. But sentencing tends to focus exclusively upon the offender – that person's incentives, punishment, deterrence, rehabilitation. In most cases the victim is not even present – the demand for pre-sentence reports to assist sentencers ensures that this is so. It is not unusual, where the matter is resolved with a guilty plea, for the victim not even to be aware that the case has been concluded. This means, incidentally, that he or she may never know what sentence was imposed, but the real loss lies in the failure publicly to acknowledge and condemn the violence. After all they have gone through, assault victims need to feel vindicated. For some this is bound up with the sentence: they want to see their assailant sent to prison. But even in serious cases the judge may have compelling 'public interest' reasons for adopting a more lenient course. This is what happened in the case of Daniel Howard, the man who broke the nose of the arresting police officer, PC Ronald Pratt (28). Unusually, Pratt, who had to have two operations and was off work for six weeks, was in court to hear Howard given a suspended sentence. We understood why the judge preferred not to send Howard to prison. He was a recidivist who had just been released after serving 15 months for another assault. The judge wanted to try a fresh approach. The unfortunate aspect of this was that there appeared no acknowledgement of the harm – the completely unjustified harm – which the victim had suffered.

These themes of denunciation and vindication are relevant even where there is no prospect of the defendant being sent to prison. This is particularly true of 'domestic' assault, where the victim's burden in bringing an assailant to court is likely to be particularly onerous. In these cases the assault is often the latest incident in a catalogue of violence and it is *this* that the victim wants acknowledged. The sentence may be incidental: what is important is that the private abuse is brought to public notice. Recognition and condemnation together bring vindication. Unfortunately the court's handling of 'domestic' and other non-stranger assault is such that, even where conviction is achieved, the violence may not be condemned. This is because the court has other purposes to fulfil. It cannot be predicted whether, in the individual case, the court's purposes match those of the victim. This is not a question which the court finds it necessary to ask. This marginalisation of the victim is inappropriate given that the criminal court is not simply responding to an offence against the sovereign authority – it is also responding to an individual wrong. The harm which the victim has suffered is of a very different order to that which we suffer collectively. The victim's marginalisation is also inappropriate given his or her role in advancing and sustaining the prosecution case, a responsibility admitted by police and prosecutors but seldom acknowledged in court.

Chapter 8

Assault, prosecution and the victim

It has been our task in this book to try to convey the reasons behind the decisions taken at each stage of the criminalisation process in respect of assault – decisions taken first by the victim, but subsequently by the police, the CPS and the court. In order to do this we have had to distinguish between assaults in different contexts, involving varying degrees of prior personal relationship, with victims who experience varying degrees of social oppression and recurring physical threat. Not all victims can ask for help, and some of those who do are unlikely to be listened to. A sampling frame which is independent of the criminal justice system – beginning with incidents before they are subject to categorisation by that system – affords a unique insight. The observer can remain sensitive to the ambiguities and uncertainties of victim stories and aware of the difficulty of arriving at a full understanding of each incident. A 'victim' may, whether as a result of shock, drink, drugs or other mental impairment, have a confused recollection of what took place, and may, either unconsciously or deliberately, misrepresent the degree of his or her own culpability. Sometimes the lifestyle of the victim may be so impenetrable that it is difficult to have any real understanding of the context of the assault. The difficulties which we as researchers encountered in penetrating some assaults may be taken as illustrative of the generally problematic nature of interpersonal violence. From the point of view of the police and the CPS there are formidable difficulties in arriving at a plausible version of what happened and, second, formidable difficulties in proving this to a court.

Although only a minority of assaults are prosecuted, these cases are useful in providing rival *accounts*: we can compare the victim's perception of the offending behaviour with the presentation of that behaviour in court. Even where there is *no* prosecution it is possible to make comparisons between victim accounts and the police perception of the event. We found that there is a problem in the definition, and so the criminalisation, of a great deal of violent behaviour. Where several people are involved and the victims can be distinguished only as those who suffer the worst injuries, it can be extremely difficult to apportion blame. Even where the violence has all been on one side, questions of provocation and precipitation arise. Some victims accept that they behaved provocatively, perhaps because they were intoxicated. But 'provocation' is itself an elastic concept. It can for example be broadened to encompass 'mouthiness' on the part of a woman towards her partner, lack of professional skill (as in a confrontation between publican and customer), or the transgression of cultural norms (where a woman acts 'above her station' in confronting a man). These were forms of provocation readily admitted, but that did not mean that these assault victims believed that the violence inflicted upon them had been justified. It was simply that they understood the reason for it.

A successful prosecution for assault demands, ideally, a blameless victim with well-defined injuries, a clearly culpable offender, and a readily accessible story. This, as we discovered, is an unusual circumstance. Christie's 'ideal victim' (vulnerable; respectable; not contributing to his or her own victimisation) is in short supply, as is his ideal offender (powerful; bad; a stranger to the victim). Most violent offenders whom the police are able to identify are known to their victim and perhaps intimately connected with him or her. Christie argues that the fact that most offenders are *not* ideal – that they are much like the rest of us – is a message which will not be listened to until crime victims are brought into such close proximity to 'their' offender that they can no longer mythologise that person; personal knowledge makes for realistic and multi-dimensional evaluation. Where the victim has no contact with the person who has done the harm he or she may need to call on various stereotypes of the offender in order to make sense of his experience – he or she may, as a result, carry an unnecessary burden of fear and incom prehension. This may be true of car thieves and burglars – their victims seldom meet them and so may well develop harsh, stereotypical images – but lack of personal knowledge of the assailant is not a problem for most assault victims. They know their assailants only too well, perhaps see them every day, and it is for this reason that readily detectable assaults can be so difficult to prosecute. Christie's message concerns the need to bridge the gulf of understanding between offenders on the one hand and victims and sentencers on the other. But assault is a special case: the problem, all too often, is one of too *great* a knowledge, too great a proximity. Victims commonly need greater protection than is afforded them by the police and courts; in other words, *more* distance from the offender, not less.

CRIMINALISATION

We have referred throughout this book to the 'criminalisation' of assault, by which we mean the various stages by which a violent act is brought within the purview of the criminal law and the perpetrator held to account for his or her actions. It is possible to break this process down in various ways, but the key steps would appear to be: reporting to the police; investigation *by* the police; prosecution; conviction; and sentence. This can be conceived as a series of filters of increasing fineness, with a substantial attrition rate at each stage. Such filtering may in many instances be appropriate, although the bald figures (see Figure 1.1, p. 13) inevitably provoke some questioning. Why, for example, do the police investigate substantially fewer assaults than are reported to them? The answer, as we have explained, has to do primarily with police assessments of each case's worth in the currency of the courts. The police response is 'purposive', to quote Sparks *et al.* (1977: 224), but not necessarily in a way commonly understood. It is no doubt true that 'crimes . . . thought (by somebody, for some reason) to be "serious" have a greater chance of being ultimately recorded' (Sparks *et al.* 1977: 224), but we have demonstrated that this observation begs a great many questions. Criminalisation of assault is *not* primarily determined by seriousness of physical injury. Nor is it determined by some other, more subjective criterion of seriousness. As we have shown, many other factors enter in and can prove overriding. The few very grave offences are routinely reported, investigated and (assuming detection) prosecuted, but apart from the very top end of the scale the relationship between seriousness and criminalisation is remarkable for the fact that there is *no* relationship, at least as far as we were able to determine.

Those factors which affect assault victims' willingness to go to the police (especially *intimacy* and *intimidation*) continue to exert their influence after the police have been alerted to the incident. In some cases, of course, the police are unable to identify the assailant, but with the exception of violence arising in pubs, clubs, or on the street, detection is not in itself the main problem. The police may be called to an assault to find victim and assailant still at the scene. But while this may make detection (or 'clear-up') straightforward, it may not assist prosecution. Assuming detection, the principal factor determining whether or not a reported assault proceeds to criminal prosecution is the victim's capacity to sustain commitment to the process. Our research demonstrates only too clearly why many assault victims are *unable* to do this. Those who have experienced 'domestic' violence may be uncertain, both at the initial stages of making a complaint and through further contact with the police, whether criminal prosecution of their assailant will meet their needs. This uncertainty compounds the police view of these women as unreliable complainants. For assault victims trapped in other kinds of continuing relationship with the assailant, for example drug user and supplier or (less obviously) a common social environment, further contact with the assailant can make it almost impossible to sustain a commitment to prosecution even where the injuries sustained have been extreme. If pursued, these very serious cases will inevitably be dealt with in the Crown Court; the associated delays add to the pressure on the victim, while police protection is likely to be inadequate in providing anything but the most tenuous sense of security.

By contrast, relatively trivial assaults may be prosecuted simply because an immediate arrest generates a prosecution momentum. Police officers will 'nourish' a complaint from a victim who has no particular animus against his assailant but who is willing to comply with the demands of the process. They will tend to respond less enthusiastically to those assault victims whose damaged status or wavering commitment renders them of little value in the currency of the courts. The nub of our argument follows from the finding that successful prosecution of assaults depends absolutely upon victims' commitment to the process; that victims have, in effect, a power of veto; and that the police, recognising the central importance of staunch victims to what they would regard as 'good process', operate their own filter whereby the hesitant complainant, the drunk, the verbally unskilled, the 'domestic', and the morally dubious are deflected from assuming full complainant status. Of course we understand the reasons for this: such victims are unlikely to withstand the rigours of the criminal process or to convince the trier of fact.

It is inevitable, given the burden of proof, and specifically given the demands which criminal prosecution places upon the victim, that reported assault should be subject to some testing by the police. We conceive this as an exercise in limitation, categorisation, and consolidation. It is, to a considerable extent, covert. In some cases the victim does not appreciate that a negative decision has been made; in others it is implied that the decision (say, not to proceed) is the victim's own; and a third possibility is that the investigation be pursued in such desultory fashion that the victim eventually withdraws. In practice police discretion is limited by a variety of constraints, both formal and informal. These include: the perceived need to respond to serious injury; victim expectations; media interest; and the supervision of senior officers. There is, inevitably, greater scope to deflect cases, and greater room for discretion generally, where the offence has low visibility.

It is hard to criticise the police for deflecting unpromising victims so that they do not assume full complainant status, or for not preparing a case file where the victim is ambivalent. Experience has taught the police that they have little chance of establishing the defendant's guilt unless they have a victim who is prepared, if necessary, to tell his or her story to a court. This is confirmed by our observation of the prosecution effort in respect of several very serious assaults. In these cases the police and the CPS, even though anticipating eventual failure, brought the assailant at least to the point of committal, only for the case to founder in the face of the victim's non-attendance or blatant non-co-operation thereafter. These cases were relatively unusual in that the police attempted, unsuccessfully as it transpired, to overcome the victim's reluctance. But the victim veto proved effective at whatever point it was decisively applied. Indeed on the basis of our evidence we would say that this veto is *100 per cent effective* in respect of assaults. So while we might criticise the police for being too eager to deflect the unsatisfactory complainant, we can hardly say that they are misguided, operationally speaking, to place such a premium upon the victim's commitment to the prosecution effort.

This is the aspect of police power which, on the basis of our research evidence, offers the severest threat to 'due process' values. The police ability to deflect what they consider unmeritorious cases greatly exceeds their ability to inculpate innocent defendants. That we should arrive at this conclusion is to some extent a reflection of our research method – a method which contrasts in certain key respects with that employed by McConville *et al.* (1991). McConville and his co-researchers studied cases which had already penetrated the system – they were already being investigated by the police. We started *outside* the justice system and so studied non-reports and non-arrests. We consider that McConville *et al.* did not take sufficient account of the police role as gate-keepers – they made little of the police capacity, and inclination, to *deflect* – while overemphasising the power of the police to mount effective case constructions. They also underestimated the role of other key decision-makers.

We have made it clear that our own research supports the proposition that the prosecution case is 'constructed'. To follow each assault through the various stages of testing enables the researcher to observe the narrowing and hardening of the original story. The difficulty in penetrating many assaults can lead, as we have described, to bizarre results. In the face of muddle and uncertainty we noted a tendency among police officers to construct cases from whatever material they had to hand. It is certainly possible, as we observed, for an initial police interpretation to harden into a serious misrepresentation. More commonly the victim's 'story' survives as the basis for the prosecution case, although shorn of as many doubts and ambiguities as possible.

This pattern can be understood by reference to the demands of the trial. Our observation of trials brought home to us the difficulties faced by the prosecution in achieving conviction on charges of assault. The prosecution has the task of presenting a convincing, coherent account of an incident which has in fact yielded more than one 'story'. This means that the criminalisation of assault is bound to be problematic. The court is likely to be offered a choice of stories – a choice which is so stark as to reflect, not the initial confusion faced by the police but two completely irreconcilable accounts of a single incident. Conviction in these circumstances may reflect the jury's belief that the alleged victim (and the police) would not have gone to the trouble to prepare a completely fabricated account, whereas the defendant is under a strong inducement to do so.

But achieving conviction for assault in the face of a rival story is still not easy. There has to be strong and convincing evidence from the victim and, in all probability, from at least one other witness. The police and the CPS understand this. That is why, where the victim's story is in doubt or his or her status damaged, prosecution is unlikely to follow. And it is in this respect that the account of the prosecution process presented by McConville *et al.* appears to us seriously misleading. Those authors' remorseless presentation of an all-powerful police is but half the story. It is evident even from their own account that much of what they say about police manipulation could be presented as reflecting the relative powerlessness of the police. As we ourselves observed, police case constructions often come to nothing. It is true that the make-up of the suspect population and of the convicted population is a 'construction', but it is not solely a police construction. Victims and witnesses make cases just as much as do the police. The police do indeed seek to build and control the prosecution case, but their power to do so is limited. There is a much more interesting tension than McConville *et al.* allow.

Finally on this theme of 'construction', we believe that to present the

CPS as subordinate to the police is a distortion of an observable working relationship. It is not accurate, in our experience, to view this in terms of the CPS rubber-stamping police decisions. Of course it is true that the police make the initial selection of cases for the prosecution. But it is not true that cases about which the police are unenthusiastic never reach the CPS, or that weak cases which the police decide to 'process' are routinely accepted. We observed many cases where the police conscientiously put together a prosecution file even though their assessment of the victim (or the offender) made them personally unenthusiastic. Nor does this pressure operate only in the direction identified by McConville *et al.*: police decisions are influenced, on a routine, everyday basis, by their understanding of CPS and court requirements. Many cases do not reach the CPS because the police realise that it would be a waste of time to put them forward. CPS policies constrain the police. There is, as we have said, a 'trickle down' effect. In our view it is by no means clear which, of the police and the CPS, is more successful in controlling the other. Each organisation has its own sphere of influence, but CPS influence upon police practice is inescapable.

ASSAULT, PROSECUTION AND THE VICTIM

A close study of assault such as we have undertaken inevitably leads one to question the purpose of criminal prosecution. If we take Reiner's analysis of the police function as our starting point, he is dismissive of the 'law enforcement' responsibilities of the police, arguing that the core mandate historically, and the key task operationally, is that of order maintenance. Specifically he argues that the law enforcement 'chimera . . . makes conduct that really should be approached as a low-level nuisance come to be assimilated within an all-encompassing omnibus cate- gory of "crime"' (Reiner 1985: 172). Reiner's thesis is that the reality of police work is at odds with the public image. The image is one of significant impact upon serious crime through detection and deterrence; the reality is that most demands made upon the police are of a peace-keeping nature. Our research does not itself challenge the validity of Reiner's argument, but it does provoke certain questions about it. These questions are of both an empirical and a theoretical kind. First, it could be argued, on our evidence, that the police are all too ready to respond to assaults as if they were merely a form of 'nuisance' or 'trouble', effectively ignoring the fact that responsibility for the violence lies exclusively with one party. What consequences flow from having the police respond in a so-called 'peace-keeping' mode rather than a law enforcement one? As Reiner himself acknowledges (1985: 199), it is open to question whether these 'peace-keeping' interventions are adequately and fairly handled. We would go further and argue that a close study of assault – and the police response to assault – reveals an emphasis upon restoring order which is purely pragmatic – and which might be defended on that basis – but which commonly fails to reflect culpability and harm. It is no doubt burdensome to treat all violent incidents as criminal acts which need to be prosecuted. But it is also a misrepresentation, for the most part, to treat them as an outbreak of 'trouble'. Assault is a violation of personal security. The victim's rights have been violated. The distinction between law enforcement and order maintenance is of questionable utility because *neither* need address that violation. What assault victims need, and deserve, is re-affirmation of their right to personal security. Neither restoration of order nor criminal prosecution of the assailant need of themselves make much contribution to this.

It remains possible, nonetheless, for public and private agendas to be satisfied in the one case. That appeared to be true of the brutal 'stranger' rape which we placed first in order of seriousness among the cases which we monitored. The victim secured an exemplary 'public' response from police and court which at the same time did much to relieve her private distress. At every step and on every level (with the possible exception of communication during the pre-trial period) she received the best 'service' that the justice system has to offer. The offender was swiftly arrested (for an unconnected burglary) and identified; at no time was her account called into question by the police; and she was treated sympathetically both in the immediate aftermath of the attack and throughout the progress of the case. One might say that this is the typical response to ferocious assaults upon unambiguously innocent victims where an offender is rapidly identified and guilt is established so conclusively that the offender and his or her legal advisers see no basis upon which to contest the charge. In other words it is a rarity. It is more usual for the victim to feel that he or she is called upon to serve *institutional* interests (Goldstein 1982; Miers 1992; Ziegenhagen 1978: 75). Even an arrest and successful prosecution may offer little to the victim: the protracted prosecution timetable, the limited extent to which victim/ assailant contact is monitored and controlled by the police, and the ultimate outcome in terms of a court-imposed sanction – each may impose further burdens or, alternatively, have no bearing upon the victim's own needs. Victim perception of the harm suffered is frequently not matched by legal definitions; the conduct of cases by the police and the presentation of these matters in court may be at odds with the victim's own account; and the sentence, if there is to be a sentence, can appear trivial or even insulting.

There have of late, both in Britain and the USA, been various attempts to improve the lot of crime victims at different stages in the justice process, whether through imposing a responsibility upon the police to keep victims informed of the progress of their case or through providing support for victims on court premises (Rock 1993). It is possible, of course, that the main purpose of these initiatives is to improve the reliability of victims as staunch complainants and witnesses (Miers 1992; McDonald 1976: 35). Such an interpretation might seem excessively cynical, but an exclusive focus upon the defendant is an abiding feature of the justice process: it would take a revolution in thought for that to be overturned. It is generally accepted that victims and other witnesses should be treated decently, but few reform initiatives can be said to amount to any more than that. The justice system is not *about* victims, any more than hospitals are about visitors.

That curiously mis-named document *The Victim's Charter* (Home Office 1990) does nothing to disturb this picture of the victim as an essential cog in the system, but a cog who is not recognised as having valued purposes in his or her own right. It states baldly that 'the public interest must come first', and concedes that in the court setting 'the convenience of individual witnesses has to be subordinate to the interests of justice'. There is no concession to the principle that the wrong suffered by the individual victim is any greater than the harm which we experience collectively. In a section headed 'Questions for the Future', it is asserted that:

> The traditional roles of the prosecutor and the court cannot readily accommodate matters which may be important to the victim but do not affect decisions on guilt or innocence and sentence.

This is consistent with the evidence of our research. It is also consistent with the theoretical models of criminal justice upon which the system rests. It has been observed that both the 'crime control' model of criminal justice and the 'due process' model, while antithetical to one another, are each consistent with a criminal justice system that is structurally and operationally insensitive to victims (Miers 1992; Zedner 1994: 1230). Concern for the interests of victims of crime, while an almost unassailable moral position, tends, as Miers puts it, to give second best to one or other of these dominating goals. 'Victim rights' are espoused by both camps, but there is no common agenda and, in reality, victim interests are marginal to both. Victims provide a stick with which to beat offenders, but the victim interest is not a dominant focus within the practice of criminal justice. We do not assign social meaning to victimisation in the same way as we do to offending. We conceive victimisation as *random* and *individual*: the real *social* significance, it is assumed, lies in the behaviour of the offender. Nor does criminal victim-isation carry much resonance from a human rights perspective: it is true that the victim's rights have been violated, but no one can quite work out what recompense should follow and to suggest that victims have *obligations* seems inappropriate given that they have suffered undeserved harm. All that leaves, it would seem, is the possibility of financial compensation.

Most commentators accept the argument that the primary respons-ibility for compensating the victim rests with the offender, while at the same time acknowledging that many cannot discharge this responsibility because they have insufficient funds, or because they are sentenced to imprisonment, or because they are never found. The extent of the state's obligation is then bound up with whatever conception we hold of the role of the state in general. It may be argued that the crimes which we suffer as a society stem from social and political decisions. A central function of the criminal law is to protect individual rights and it is for this reason that compensation for the victims of violent crime is properly regarded as part of the state's responsibility (Ashworth 1986). Others would argue that the payment of compensation represents an awkward grafting on of the restitutive principle to the essentially punitive frame-work of the criminal law (Zedner 1994: 1239).

Miers refers to the compensation initiatives which began in the 1960s as the birth of 'victimology', leading to the emergence of victims of violence as 'an identifiable and coherent group, with evident political potential' (Miers 1978: 51). That potential, if it ever existed, has not been realised, even if criminal injuries compensation is now reasonably well established. In fact it remains on an *ex gratia* basis and has recently been reduced in scope. The government's statement when introducing the scheme expressly denied an obligation towards crime victims, it being asserted that the CICB was based on 'the more practical ground . . . that although the Welfare State helps victims of many kinds of misfortune, it does nothing for the victims of crimes of violence as such' (White Paper, *Compensation of Victims of Crimes of Violence* (Cmnd 2323 of 1964)).

While a strong moral case can be made for the provision of state compensation, it is an inevitable weakness of this mechanism that it does not form part of the justice process but is instead a 'welfare' measure targeted at a heterogeneous victim population. This means that crime victims are equated with other groups placing financial demands upon the state – the poor, the unemployed, the old, and the handicapped (see, for example, Fattah 1986: *prologue*). There is also concern lest the costs of this provision escalate beyond the state's ability to pay. Certainly the level of applications, and of awards, has risen substantially,[1] while there is continual pressure on the government to extend the scope of the scheme.

The question of state financial compensation is a matter of secondary importance for most assault victims. Many, as we have seen, choose not to report the incident to the police and so are ineligible for any award. Others are not sufficiently injured to qualify. Some may not be informed of the possibility of making a claim, and a fourth group may welcome compensation but still regard it as a side issue. Because we are concerned with the criminal prosecution of violent acts these 'welfare' provisions are of peripheral concern to us here. Compensation may, on one conception, be owed by the state to its citizens, but that form of justice is what we call 'welfare'. Criminalisation has the potential to deliver justice to victims as well as to offenders. The provision of state compensation is incidental to that process.

The predominant purpose of criminal proceedings is to declare public disapproval of the offender's conduct (Ashworth 1986). This is done by means of public trial and conviction and the imposition of a penal sanction. Blackstone (1778) drew the distinction between public and private wrongs as follows:

> Private wrongs, or civil injuries, are an infringement or privation of the civil rights which belong to individuals, considered merely as individuals: public wrongs, or crimes and misdemeanours, are a breach and a violation of the public rights and duties, due to the whole community, considered as a community, in its social aggregate capacity.

This statement has been criticised on the basis that the distinction which it promotes is untenable: all offences affect the community and all affect individuals (Austin 1885, cited in Ashworth 1986), but Blackstone's point, as elucidated by Ashworth, is that in the case of more serious crimes the private wrong is swallowed up in the public. Certainly the interests of the victim are subordinated to, or subsumed into, the interests of the state. Ashworth's view is that the victim ought, as one citizen, to have his or her interests represented by the state: as a central figure in that particular offence the victim should not be neglected. Thus the police should inform victims of the progress of their case; victims should be informed about the state compensation scheme; the police should obtain and prosecutors should present details of a victim's injury or loss so as to provide the basis for the making of a compensation order. That said, Ashworth contends that criminal as distinct from civil liability is distinguishable on the basis of *gravity* and *intention*. The fact that the offender has deliberately chosen to do harm creates a more widespread fear and insecurity (Nozick 1974, cited in Ashworth 1986). Accordingly, argues Ashworth (1986), the victim

> has no right to consent to the infliction of most serious injuries and some other acts; no right to veto a prosecution, to demand a prosecution or to commute or demand a sentence; no right even to be consulted about the decision to prosecute or choice of sentence: these are all state decisions, to be taken upon public interest principles. The victim's rights at all these stages should be those of any other citizen, although there are good reasons for ensuring that the victim is kept informed about the progress of the case and about the general reasons for decisions taken upon it, and decisions not to prosecute should be open to challenge.

Ashworth considers what should happen where the victim does not want the offender to be prosecuted and his conclusion, just as one might expect given the other elements of his argument, is that in principle the victim's wishes should be subordinated to the public interest. He acknowledges that the central role of victims in providing evidence gives them *de facto* power to frustrate some prosecutions, but he argues that in principle the wishes of the individual victim should not be determinative.

Ashworth's is a normative statement. But our research demonstrates that *in practice* where the victim does not wish to see an assailant prosecuted (for whatever reason) his or her wishes prevail. This is anticipated by the police. As we have seen, the police do not respond to 'crime'; they respond to 'complaints'. In other words, their response is entirely dependent upon the victim's commitment to criminalisation. If there is no complaint, the police will take no action – even in respect of very serious assaults. It has been suggested that this 'reactive' approach to determining which crimes should be investigated enhances 'dominion' in that the police are responding to the will of the victim (Braithwaite and Pettit 1990: 112). By responding to complaints, the argument runs, the police implicitly render themselves accountable to the community. This limits their discretion in that they are not simply acting on the basis of their own prejudices against individuals or groups whom they might wish to target.[2] In fact it does not seem to us that the 'dominion' argument can be applied to the prosecution of assault. It is difficult to imagine any circumstance *less* productive of 'dominion' than that of being deterred from pursuing a complaint against one's assailant upon pain of further violence.

Even if it were true that 'dominion' is enhanced through the police focus upon the complaint, we observe a striking inconsistency within the criminalisation process between the early stages of arrest, charge and prosecution and, thereafter, the processes of trial and sentence which are all too faithful to the offence against society model. In cases of assault the police respond to complaints rather than crimes because they know they have little chance of establishing the defendant's guilt unless they have a victim who is prepared, if necessary, to tell his or her story to a court. But this is itself inconsistent with a view of crime as an offence against the sovereign authority; it is also inconsistent with the marginal role ascribed to victims thereafter. One might have thought, if an 'offence against society' model were in operation, that this would apply to every stage of the proceedings (in which case the police would respond to *offences* rather than to *complaints*); but it does not seem to do so. In fact there are two models in operation, complainant-oriented at the police end and 'offence against society'-oriented at the court end.

We are interested in this disjunction because it is largely unrecognised. It is commonly observed that the justice process is an arduous one for many crime victims, and that their interests tend to be neglected within it, but what tends not to be acknowledged is the extent to which normative accounts of criminal justice as *state* prosecution are overridden, at least in respect of violent offences, by a pragmatic acceptance on the part of the police and the CPS of their absolute dependence upon victim commitment to the process. Ashworth argues that the victim's wishes should be subordinated to the public interest in matters of prosecution policy. Actual practice is very different. If a theoretical model departs too far from empirical reality, either the model itself needs to be revised or else *the practice* of criminal justice should be modified so that it bears some relationship to the normative account.

One of the assault victims whom we interviewed, Amanda Britton (53), expressed the view that it should be the police, rather than the victim, who bore responsibility for initiating prosecution. This, she suggested, would do much to meet the victim's need for support and security at the point when an assault was reported. Part of the burden would be lifted. This proposal, or some variant of it, is most commonly made in the context of 'domestic' assault. For example, it has been asserted that an arrest should automatically be made whenever an assault has taken place, regardless of the wishes of the injured party. Only by this means can violence against women be converted to an issue automatically necessitating public intervention and women be guaranteed protection from further attack.

(Faragher 1985)

Changes along these lines have already been implemented in some US states in the context of domestic violence. How far this has achieved the protection (as against the further victimisation) of women who report domestic assault is still the subject of debate (Morley and Mullender 1992).

The same argument can be applied to assaults which do not take place in a domestic context. But, as in the domestic sphere, there would remain formidable practical difficulties in seeking to implement such a moral imperative. The case studies referred to in this book give some indication of the vital role played by the victim as witness. The probative burden cannot be satisfied without this evidence. Even were the alleged victim *compelled* to give evidence, such testimony would be of limited value. Also, the practice of 'compelling' witnesses might be considered morally dubious in itself. We are ourselves sceptical as to the practicability of a mandatory prosecution policy. Certainly if attempts were made to move in this direction a greatly improved system of support for victim witnesses would need to be set up. Victim Support has introduced Victim/Witness in Court schemes at many Crown Courts, following the success of seven pilot projects. The report of these experiments (Raine and Smith 1991; Rock 1993) suggests a satisfactory 'take-up' of the support offered. This therefore might form part of a more comprehensive support network. There would also be need for more effective police protection. Taken together, these steps might go some way towards overcoming the tendency for assault victims to withdraw their co-operation with the prosecuting authorities.

A second possible approach to resolving the inconsistency which we have identified would be to attempt in some other way to compensate victims for the pains of the criminalisation process. They might, for example, be granted more influence upon the *outcome* of that process. That is what seems to be anticipated by Miers when he identifies 'the shift . . . of responsibility for significant elements of the implementation of criminal justice police, from the public to the private sector'. As a result, says Miers, the Home Office multi-agency approach to crime prevention now depends heavily upon the exercise of private responsibility in preventing crime. Accordingly, 'we may expect correspondingly stronger claims that victims be given rights in the determination of criminal justice decisions' (Miers 1992).

In fact, as we have described, assault victims *do* in a manner of speaking take criminal justice decisions. But they lose all authority, even influence, by the time their case comes to court. It is doubtful whether even the introduction of victim impact statements would do much to alter the offender focus of criminal proceedings (McDonald 1976: 31). This is because criminal justice is conceived as a response to a violation of a social norm rather than, primarily, as a response to harm done to an individual. The symbolic purpose is dominant. Supposed utilitarian justifications for court penalties are for the most part rationalisations – it is the symbolic purpose that matters. 'Justice' is an intangible – it belongs to our 'symbolic world of meanings' (Berger and Luckmann 1966, quoted in Bussman 1992). Criminal law is an important part of this. We should not label it as irrational; it is as rational as a symbolic message can be (Bussman 1992).

Arnold has similarly argued that we should not be surprised that there is little similarity between the ideals of the law and what courts actually do (Arnold 1969). This is because it is part of the function of law to give recognition to ideals which represent the exact opposite of established conduct. Most legal complications arise from the necessity of pretending to do one thing while actually doing another. Legal principles are supposed to control society, because such an assumption is necessary to the logic of the dream-world created by law, but the observer should constantly keep in mind that the function of law is not so much to guide society as to comfort it. This does not mean that criminal sanctions do not matter. Most present-day commentators would accept in some form the Durkheimian thesis that punishment is necessary in order to maintain moral order and legal authority; failure to punish violations of the *conscience collectif* undermines social morality and demoralises citizens (Garland 1990: 59). State punishment is a sign that the authorities are in control, that crime is an aberration, and that the conventions which govern social life retain their vitality (*ibid.*). Dahrendorf (1985: 20, quoted in Garland 1990: 60) likewise argues that sanctions have to have some force if they are to have this system-maintaining effect. Specifically he argues that some sanctions employed against young and first offenders have become so 'emasculated' that they have contributed to the collapse of the authoritative social order. This weakening of sanctions has led to the anomic consequences predicted by Durkheim.

The view that law is a moralising symbol provides one explanation as to why criminal justice is unlikely to place much emphasis upon remedying the harm suffered by the individual victim. The retributive paradigm focuses on the violation of norms and values. There is not much scope for argument about harm, or about remedy, within a system whose principal function is to excoriate the most grossly anti-social acts. The 'justice' in criminal justice is expressed through the infliction of an appropriate measure of pain. The relationship between victim and offender has been defined by the charge; there is no scope for exploring what might be a fair outcome as between the two of them – neither victim nor offender has the status of being a party to the proceedings. At the same time one may discern continued demand and, some would say, expectation that the criminal courts deliver individualised justice (Friedman 1985). Friedman argues that "a general expectation of justice" is replacing the former low expectation of criminal proceedings. This, he suggests, produces many problems, not least for lawyers themselves since they know they cannot deliver what is being asked of them.

The symbolism of law enforcement tends primarily to be acknowledged where there is a doubt (at least in some people's eyes) as to whether the behaviour in question should be criminalised at all. Those who argue *in favour* of criminalisation tend to do so not on the basis of individual remedy but on the ground that law, in condemning a particular type of behaviour, shapes public opinion. This can be seen in relation to 'domestic' assault. Edwards and Halpern (1992) assert that:

> the criminal law serves an important symbolic and denunciatory function in conveying to the aggressor and to society that such violence will not be tolerated . . . The symbolic nature of the law – its declaratory and denunciatory functions – is important in shaping climates of opinion. The criminal law is after all a normative statement. It sets the boundaries of acceptable behaviour. It is a statement of how people ought to behave and what will happen if they do not.

These commentators argue that if the criminal law is not enforced in respect of this group of assaults a 'message' is conveyed that domestic violence is not worth bothering about. The law's response is important both in its impact upon other agencies and in helping to create a climate of opinion in which domestic violence is regarded unambiguously as a criminal act meriting public censure and sanction.

In fact the symbolism of the law, specifically in relation to assault, seems to us more complicated than this. The public presentation of assault in, say, the magistrates' court is a low-key affair. That is not to say that it is bereft of symbolism, but one needs to observe the proceedings carefully in order to assess the symbolic content. The 'message' that is conveyed is not necessarily one of abhorrence of male violence inflicted upon women. It can equally be that this is a trivial transgression to which the court sees fit to give only fleeting attention. Or the message may be that the victim is as culpable as his or her assailant. The symbolism of the lower courts (or indeed of the Crown Court, when dealing with offences at the bottom of the tariff) can threaten the status of *all* non-professional participants, victims and defendants alike. In short, it is not enough to bring cases to court – that is no guarantee that the desired symbolic message will be conveyed. It follows that there can be no neat separation of the individual and the symbolic. For all but the most heinous, high-profile offence, the symbolism of the court process is inescapably bound up with the treatment of the individual victim. 'Domestic' violence offers an easy illustration, although we would contend that the point is valid across all violence prosecutions. The symbolism is not necessarily that which the division of lay actors into the two classes of 'victim' and 'offender' might lead one to imagine. Courts will not convey the *desired* symbolic message unless they demon-strate within each case that they are concerned about the experience of the individual victim. If that does not happen, the symbolic message will be rather different – a punitive message in respect of both parties, perhaps.

Discussion of the role of victims within criminal proceedings has tended to focus upon the scope for incorporating some form of civil remedy either within or alongside criminal justice (Campbell 1984; Davis 1992: *passim*). Alternatively, the case is argued for some form of mediated encounter. In fact assault victims are in general less likely than victims of other offences to welcome a meeting with the offender in their case (O'Brien 1986). Edward Jones (25) provides one example of this. He had no unanswered questions; he was prepared to accept that some people do react violently in these circumstances; his injuries were public and self-evident; his own behaviour was not under scrutiny; he preferred to 'file' the incident. At the same time the Christie insights did receive some support from our study – occasionally from surprising sources. For example, Walter Drobny (32), who had been 'mugged' outside his home and who as a result was fearful of venturing out, was firm in his wish to meet his assailants and to confront them with the harm which they had done. This suggests that there is a distinction to be made between inchoate fear of unknown attackers and a wish to confront one's assailant in a controlled situation. The same point was made by the two student nurses, Louise Duke and her friend (69), assaulted by a stranger wield-ing a stick as they walked home after an evening out. They both expressed a wish to meet their attacker, provided of course that they felt protected. The incident was totally unprovoked and they wanted to discover what lay behind it.

The most thoughtful response to our question concerning whether the victim would like to meet his assailant came from Julian Davies (52), the young man 'mugged' in the St Paul's district of Bristol where he (reluctantly) found himself living. Asked for his feelings about his assailant, he replied:

> I don't feel outraged . . . I would rather speak to him and ask him why he did it. At the moment, the person who hit me is just an object to me . . . that's why I would like to meet him . . . I would like to explain to him that it's not a nice thing to do. I believe there are some people – their whole life is like that . . . I mean, they're just going to go on doing it. It's not as if I've got no understanding of the motives. The fact that I'm a victim is because I live here – and I don't want to live here. I would like him to hear it from my point of view . . . I don't necessarily think a spell in prison would make him a better person. My attitude to him is . . . I don't know him.

So Davies was prepared to think of his assailant as a person in his own right, with his own problems. He did not simply label him as a criminal:

> It wasn't a serious assault – it wasn't a terrible thing. But I don't *like* it, and I don't think it's the right way to carry on. I'd like him to try to understand that from my point of view. He might have thought that I was just a white person going through St Paul's . . . I don't know what he thought.

Despite the above, the dominant impression from our study was one of victims wishing to distance themselves from their assailant and put the incident behind them. In so far as they sought confrontation, this tended to be a public confrontation such as, they imagined, might be achieved in court, with the offender being brought publicly to account for what he or she had done. It may be of course that the very availability of public prosecution undermines people's capacity to deal with conflict, including interpersonal violence (Christie 1977). Those most habituated to the system are the ones least likely to see any feasible alternative. Three of the assault victims whom we interviewed were policemen, or ex-policemen. One of them, Jonathan Musgrove (45), continued to frequent the same pub as the man who had broken his jaw. His assailant had pleaded guilty to an ABH charge and been fined, but it appeared that this public outcome had provided little in the way of private resolution for the two principal actors. As Musgrove described the situation:

> Three times out of four on a Sunday that particular person will be in that pub, though not sat anywhere near us. He's made no effort to speak to me and I've made no effort to speak to him. He's been arrested and dealt with as the court sees fit; my opinion as to whether he should have been fined greater or as to whether a compensation order should have been made is irrelevant. The case has been dealt with. He's got no reason to speak to me, as he knows he was in the wrong, otherwise he wouldn't have pleaded guilty.

So despite certain misgivings concerning the conduct of the case, Musgrove expressed himself satisfied with public acknowledgement of his assailant's guilt. Would some kind of mediated confrontation have achieved a better outcome? No doubt some people want to convey whatever it is they feel as a result of the assault; others would prefer not. We are dealing here with the two dimensions of confrontation/non-confrontation (or acknowledgement/non-acknowledgement) and, second, of public/ private resolution. Courts are public, but so are some 'tribal' models of dispute resolution. Mediated encounters in our culture are almost invariably private and do not necessarily reflect the victim's interests or agenda (Davis 1992). We are loath to suggest that any one model should, necessarily, be preferred. What is readily apparent is that both public prosecution and mediated encounter can each in their own way impose considerable burdens upon the victim – burdens often not attended by any compensatory reward. As these things are handled at the moment, it is doubtful whether victims benefit greatly from either. All one can say is that one set of processes is familiar while the other is not.

Recent attempts to develop mediation and reparation programmes in the UK have had limited success, thereby confirming the intractability of our criminal justice institutions and demonstrating the remarkable ease with which vested interests in the penal system marginalise ideas which threaten basic assumptions (Davis 1992: *passim*). Partly as a consequence of this failure to integrate mediatory and reparative initiatives into the justice process one observes a growing tendency to argue that criminal justice should be delivered in two strands – on the one hand public denunciation, fulfilling a symbolic purpose and catering for the worst criminal acts, and on the other the communicative and reparative, reflecting the value attached to rational communication in the aftermath of dispute (Bussman 1992).

This argument is superficially attractive, but our observation of assault prosecutions leads us to conclude that it is mistaken. Of course it is true that the interests of the victim may diverge from the interests of the various professional actors within criminal justice. But one should not drive too substantial a wedge between so-called 'public' and 'private' interests. Private citizens have interests which are grounded in their citizenship as much as in their individual personal identity. During the course of our research we spoke to assault victims who wanted the circumstances of their assault to receive a public airing. Their reason for wanting this was partly their sense that a crime had been committed – they thought the law should take its course; and partly, also, they appeared to want their assailant brought to account. They wanted public acknowledgement that they had suffered a wrong. We understand of course that this aspiration may be based upon a misconception about what actually goes on in court – at best boredom and bathos, at worst a misrepresentation of facts, distortion of victim accounts and humiliation of the witness under cross-examination. But it nonetheless suggests that victims have certain needs – for support, reassurance and vindication – which *can* be met by the public procedures of the criminal courts, even if in fact the trial process is deficient in many of these 'public' aspects.

It is not only restitution or other forms of reparation which should be seen as meeting the needs of the individual crime victim. The victim has an interest in punishment. The symbolic purposes of the law have meaning for that person as well as for the rest of society; the definition of a certain form of behaviour as criminal and the consequent public condemnation and punishment of the perpetrator can reassure the victim that he or she has public recognition and support. If one were entirely to privatise the response to assault, permitting the harmed person merely the status of a civil complainant, the law might become more sensitive to the scope for reparative action by the offender; the victim might have greater opportunity to tell his or her story. But this would also have the effect of redefining the true nature of what had taken place, reducing it to the status of a private quarrel. From the victim's point of view that might be at least as much a misrepresentation as any which he or she is likely to suffer, at present, in the courtroom.

Research method

We approached victims either directly in the Accident and Emergency Department of the Bristol Royal Infirmary, or on the wards, or at out-patient clinics, or by letter. By these means we gained access to ninety-two assault victims. In eighty-eight of these cases we conducted a full interview with the victim and, where the matter was reported to the police, we interviewed the officer in the case. Where the case went to court we endeavoured to attend all court hearings. In this way we were able to gain a complete picture of the factors which determined, at each successive stage, whether an assault was criminalised.

The two *main* strategies employed in approaching victims were by means of a letter or, alternatively, through attendance at the Accident and Emergency Department. During the period October 1990–February 1991 we contacted (by means of a letter signed by the Consultant Head of Department) batches of potential informants drawn from those patients who registered at the A & E Department giving the cause of their injury as assault. During this period we also contacted by letter a small number of assault victims who were receiving out-patient treatment under the supervision of Dr Jon Shepherd at the Bristol Dental Hospital. A total of 292 letters were sent. Of these, 199 produced no response; twenty-six produced a negative response; nine were returned unopened; and fifty-eight produced a positive response. Of the fifty-eight people who expressed an initial willingness to talk to us, fifty responded to our follow-up letter or phone-call and were interviewed. (One of these interviewees was found to have suffered two separate assaults within the space of a week, so she gave rise to two separate 'cases'.)

It is evident that we suffered a high failure rate in respect of potential informants whom we approached by letter. Assault victims who have no fixed address, or who in general do not read or reply to letters, cannot be secured by this means. That said, we achieved an excellent response through our *attendance* at the hospital (see below), managing to secure interviews with some, such as habitual drug users, who might be expected to elude a research study of this kind.

This second strategy involved attendance in the A & E Department on a number of nights during the period October 1990 – May 1991. The nights chosen were Thursday, Friday or Saturday, in recognition of the fact that these were likely to produce a great many assaults. We designated this our 'Hospital Attendance' sample and we included in it victims who were approached while receiving in-patient treatment. In the case of this latter group we were alerted to their presence on the wards by reception staff in the A & E Department or by Dr Shepherd. By these means we approached a further fifty-two victims, forty-nine of whom agreed to be interviewed. Of these forty-nine, sixteen subsequently declined or did not respond to further contact, leaving thirty-three who were actually interviewed. In addition we followed a further four cases even though we were unable to have more than a brief conversation with the victim (who, in each instance, was very severely injured). We obtained five cases by other means. Of these, three were University of Bristol students and the other two were identified in the course of interviews with other informants.

In total, therefore, we followed ninety-two victims (or ninety-three cases). Following our initial contact, and usually within a few days or weeks of the assault, we spent approximately an hour with each victim, usually in his or her own home, discussing as fully as possible the circumstances of the assault, the victim's attitude towards criminalisation, and his or her reflections on what had happened and its implications in the longer term. The interviews were loosely structured and were in almost all cases tape-recorded and selectively transcribed. A few interviews were carried out on the ward and were not tape-recorded. These were subsequently written up from notes.

We encountered rather more reported than unreported assaults, the picture being confused somewhat by the fact that in some instances where the victim claimed to have gone to the police no crime report had been made out. In each of the fifty-three cases which had been recorded by the police, even if only on their daily incident 'log', we interviewed the officer principally concerned. Where different officers had played key roles at different stages in the conduct of the case we tried to interview all those involved. (The most police interviews which we conducted in respect of a single case was four.) We talked to officers, often at some length, about their role in the case, examining the decisions taken. As with our victim interviews these conversations were tape-recorded and we then provided a full thematic summary, including selective transcription. All this was achieved thanks to the generous assistance of the Avon and Somerset police.

In the twenty-six cases which involved at least one appearance at court we attended all the various hearings, including committal proceedings. We took full notes and recorded the charge before the court, the plea, and the offence of which the offender was ultimately convicted. If there was a trial, we attended throughout, noting especially the prosecution and defence cases and their relationship to our prior understanding of the incident giving rise to the trial; the role of the victim as witness; the plea in mitigation; and the relationship between the outcome and the prior expectations of victim and police.

All our interviews with victims were completed by 30 June 1991 and the bulk of the interviews with police officers were also completed by that time. Our fieldwork was completed in January 1992 when we concluded our court observation.

The cases

These accounts represent, broadly, the stories told to us by victims, although we have occasionally included material which was disclosed during discussions with a police officer in the case. Where there appeared to us to be doubt about the circumstances of the incident we have acknowledged this. The cases are presented in descending order of seriousness according to our own ranking, with case 1 being the most serious, and so on.

1. **Miranda Hooper**, a teacher in her forties, was the victim of a violent sexual attack by a stranger who had gained entry to her house on a pretext. Returning to her house one night Hooper encountered a young man, Jason Madden, who claimed to have been injured and asked to come in and wash. Thinking that he cut 'a pathetic figure', Hooper let him in and directed him to the kitchen sink. Almost immediately Madden picked up a kitchen knife and threatened Hooper with it, demanding that she allow him to have intercourse with her. Hooper put up a determined struggle against her assailant who, having made several unsuccessful attempts at rape, forced her upstairs to her bedroom. There, in a prolonged and vicious attack, he raped her and forced her to submit to other sexual acts. Eventually Hooper managed to break away and ran downstairs screaming. Her screams at last alerted the occupants of her basement flat, who came upstairs to investigate. On their appearance the intruder fled.

2. **Matthew Saunders** had an umbrella thrown at him, spear fashion, catching him in the eye and breaking the bone at the back of the eye, compressing his brain. He immediately and irreparably lost the sight of that eye. The incident arose from a three-cornered relationship in which Saunders' girlfriend of 15 years had formed a

relationship with a Michael Addis, who lived next door to Saunders. One evening, when he had been drinking heavily, Saunders went round to remonstrate with Addis and actually began breaking his front door down in an attempt to confront him and his former girlfriend. Addis, who is alcoholic and was in his habitual state of intoxication, ran down the stairs towards the glass-panelled front door, snatching up an umbrella which he then launched through the partly broken glass of the door.

3. **Patrick Dashwood** and three friends, northerners working temporarily in Bristol, were badly injured in the course of an attack in the city centre. An argument developed when one of Dashwood's companions, Mike Platt, was 'chatting up' three girls in a car near to the entrance of the pub where they had all been drinking. One of these girls happened to be the girlfriend of a bouncer from the pub, a Mr Brenton. On noticing the encounter Brenton approached and persuaded or dragged Platt from the car. Following an acrimonious exchange Brenton returned to the pub. Almost immediately a group of young men, all of them thought to be bouncers, ran up the street. Three of the four northerners were then subjected to a concentrated and prolonged attack. They were knocked to the ground and repeatedly kicked while unconscious. The man most seriously injured spent three days in intensive care and a second victim has since suffered recurring epileptic fits.

4. **David Freeman**, aged 21, spent much of his early life in children's homes. He subsequently became a heroin addict and served a prison term. A few days before this assault Freeman had agreed to act as a dealer on behalf of one of the St Paul's drugs gangs. Suspecting him of pocketing some of the proceeds, four gang members went to the flat where Freeman was 'working' in order to exact summary justice and secure the return of their money. Over the next few hours Freeman was subjected to a sustained attack with many refinements, including scalding, a partial drowning, stabbing with various implements and beatings with a baseball bat. His arm was broken in two places and he had bruises and burns over much of his body. Freeman was then driven to a former address where he claimed to have money. Once there he managed to free himself and raise the alarm. The gang fled upon the arrival of the police.

5. **Louise Purnell** was subjected to a savage and prolonged attack by her partner, in the course of which she received internal injuries as well as extensive cuts and bruises all over her body. Her partner, Jason Adebayo, held Purnell captive in their home for some 24 hours. Eventually Purnell managed to escape to the house of an aunt who lives nearby. The aunt reported the attack to the police before taking Purnell to hospital for treatment.

6. **Timothy Paxman** is a young man in his mid-twenties with ten years of heroin addiction behind him and no realistic prospect of breaking the habit. He was viciously assaulted by his supplier, to whom he owed £50. This man, with an associate, first destroyed Paxman's car with blows from a baseball bat and then employed the same weapon on Paxman, breaking both his arms. He also cut Paxman about the face with a Stanley knife. The police were called by a third party who reported the attack upon the car.

7. **Michael Fleming** is a man of powerful physique who dresses in the manner of the 1960s biker he once was. He had agreed to tow away a neighbour's car from a street in St Paul's, where it had broken down. While attaching the tow rope Fleming, who had a friend with him, left his van blocking the street. A car containing two young men drove up behind him and the driver of this car sounded his horn fiercely. An argument developed and this was concluded only when the driver mounted the pavement at great speed and shot away. With the tow rope fixed, Fleming drove slowly off; his friend was at the wheel of the car on tow. As he turned a corner Fleming put his head out of the window of his van, suspecting that there was some problem with the towing. At that moment he was hit very hard over the head with a brick. Completely disorientated, Fleming got out of his van and wandered dazedly around, his face a mask of blood. A police van quickly arrived at the scene and an ambulance was called. Fleming had suffered a severe skull fracture.

8. **Steven Clutton**, aged 18, had been enjoying a night out in the city centre with a group of male friends when, at 2 a.m., he was attacked. As a result of the beating and kicking he received, Clutton's skull was fractured and his jaw broken. His memories of the incident are confused, but he recalls going to the help of one of his friends who had been set upon in the street by a gang of perhaps a dozen youths. One of these youths punched Clutton's friend and then, when

Clutton intervened, the group turned their aggression on him. Clutton's other friends ran off but Clutton was knocked to the ground and kicked where he lay. It is not known who called the police but when Clutton was found his attackers had disappeared.

9. **Michael McTear** was stabbed in the stomach while drinking in a pub. McTear, aged 23, had spent a Sunday lunch-time in a pub which he regularly frequents. According to McTear an argument developed among a group of drinkers behind him and when he turned to see what was going on he became involved and was almost immediately stabbed. Feeling pain, but unaware of the severity of his injury, McTear attempted to walk away but fell to the floor. An ambulance was called and McTear was rushed to hospital where his life was saved by an emergency operation.

10. **Andrew Barker**, a young man with many criminal associates and, almost certainly, a criminal lifestyle, was leaving a notorious city centre pub late one evening in the company of a severely inebriated woman friend and her small dog. A taxi had been called to take Barker and the girl home, but when the woman (and her dog) got into the taxi a fierce row developed between her and the taxi driver. Barker became involved and a scuffle ensued, in the course of which Barker felt a severe blow to his chest. He had in fact been stabbed and his lung had been punctured. The taxi drove off; police and an ambulance were called by bystanders.

11. **Howard Henderson**, a man in his forties, was returning home from an illegal drinking club in St Paul's when he was was attacked in the street as he waited for a lift. A car containing three men drew up and the occupants asked Henderson if he could supply them with drugs. Henderson (who says that he does not deal in drugs) was in conversation with these men when a youth, known to him by sight, approached and accused Henderson of trespassing on his 'patch'. The car drove off and the argument between Henderson and the youth flared into violence. The youth produced a gun but Henderson managed to wrest this from him and throw it away. Henderson was gaining the upper hand when someone came to his opponent's aid. Thereupon the tables were turned; Henderson was knocked to the ground and given a severe kicking. His jaw was broken in several places. A passer-by called an ambulance. Henderson's attacker also sought hospital treatment for a cut foot and it was this which

led to his identification and subsequent arrest. (He gave his correct name and address and was filmed on the hospital security video.)

12. **Mike Cowan**, aged 34, is a heroin addict who himself has convictions for violence. Early one evening, as Cowan was taking his young son to catch a bus home to his mother (Cowan's ex-partner), he became involved in 'banter' with four youths. Cowan, who described himself as having been 'stoned' at the time, cannot remember clearly who initiated the physical violence. Blows were struck on either side before Cowan was knocked to the ground. At this all four youths laid into him with their feet but desisted on the intervention of a middle-aged woman passer-by, who grabbed one of the assailants and verbally abused the others. Cowan's hip and arm were broken in the attack, which he chose not to report to the police.

13. **Patrick Mangan**, a recently appointed publican, was assaulted by a customer. He was called to a disturbance in the bar and, this having been contained, invited one of the protagonists – a young man with whom he had previously had some trouble – to talk over the incident in the pub lobby. Mangan was in the process of banning, or threatening to ban, the youth when he was struck on the side of the head. His assailant then pulled Mangan's shirt half over his head and tugged him out into the car park. Mangan fell to the ground, seriously injuring his knee. He was given a severe kicking to the body before being rescued by bar staff. Mangan's leg was fractured in three places, necessitating a graft from his hip to repair the bone damage around the knee. He also suffered a broken finger and various cuts and bruises.

14. **Tom Robinson** was attacked in the street on New Year's Eve as he made his way to a Bristol bail hostel. He had been committed to the hostel that day from Wells magistrates' court, where he was charged with assaulting his wife. A man in his sixties, Robinson has a drink problem and although a condition of his bail was that he should not drink he had, by his own account, had a few drinks in the course of his bus journey to Bristol. He can remember nothing of the attack. He told us that he had the impression that he was taken to hospital in a police van, but he only fully regained consciousness in hospital, where he found himself wrapped in foil, suffering from hypothermia. He had suffered deep gashes to his head and right arm, a

bruised leg and a broken jaw. His wallet, which he claimed had contained £100, was missing. After five nights in hospital Robinson was released to the bail hostel. He reported the missing wallet to the police.

15. **Philip Harriman**, a retired sergeant major aged 66, was attacked by a close neighbour, Richard Baron. Harriman, a widower, and Baron's wife Christine had developed a close relationship. According to Harriman they had agreed to end this but Baron disbelieved their intention. On the night of the attack Harriman was spending a convivial evening at home with friends when Baron telephoned, inviting him round, apparently to talk things over. Harriman agreed, uncertain what to expect. Of the attack itself he has no clear recollection. It seems that he and Baron were having some discussion in the front room when Baron became violent, battering Harriman with a stool. At some point Christine intervened and Harriman managed to stagger back home, where his friends put him to bed. The next day his GP sent him to hospital where he was found to have a broken collar bone, three damaged ribs, internal bleeding and a broken nose.

16. **Walter Bristow** was lying low in St Paul's following the robbery of a restaurant. He is a heavy drug user and had just spent the weekend crashed out on cocaine when he was accosted in the street by a former prison acquaintance. This man accused Bristow of having a relationship with his girlfriend. He forced Bristow into the hallway of a block of flats, then knocked him out with a single blow. Bristow's injuries (a black eye, broken jaw and extensive bruising) suggested that he must then have been kicked as he lay unconscious. When he regained consciousness his attacker had left. Bristow was able to make his way to hospital on foot, with the help of a friend.

17. **George Griffin** is well-known in his locality as a wheeler-dealer and volatile, heavy drinking rogue. He has an extensive criminal record, mainly arising from his habit of 'shopping after hours' – burglary – and from his tendency to engage in well-lubricated physical violence upon his ex-wife, the police, or anyone else who crosses his path. On this occasion Griffin was given a beating as he was leaving his local pub. He sustained a badly broken cheekbone plus other minor injuries. Griffin thinks that he was attacked by two

or three men and though he was not able to identify them he believes – not implausibly in view of his local reputation – that he was singled out for these attentions.

18. **Gary Atkinson** was the victim of a fierce and prolonged beating in the toilet of a pub in the city centre where he is a regular, high-profile, customer. There had, it seems, been no immediate provocation but the attack followed on a history of ill-feeling between Atkinson and his assailant. In the course of the attack Atkinson suffered facial bruising, a flattened nose, multiple cuts to the nose and mouth, the loss of two teeth and deep bruising to the body. Onlookers attempted to intervene but the onslaught ended only when the press of bodies in the gents effectively prevented further blows being struck.

19. **Michael Tapper**, a divorced man of 51, suffered a hairline skull fracture when he was assaulted by a man called Dave Ewing, the husband of a woman with whom Tapper had been having a relationship. Tapper, the manager of a DIY store, was confronted by Ewing one Sunday morning in the empty car park of his shop. Tapper was in the act of closing his car sun-roof when Ewing approached and kicked the car door with some force, causing Tapper to fall and strike his head on the ground or on some part of the car. What happened next is not clear, but it seems that Ewing struck Tapper several blows before driving off. Tapper managed to stagger into his shop and alert his assistant. An ambulance (called by Ewing) arrived shortly afterwards.

20. **Timothy Cooper**, a pub landlord, was the victim of a 'glassing' by one of his customers during a busy, noisy evening. Cooper's young assailant, Roy Camp, was sitting at the bar with a friend. They were part of a large group of rowdy customers. Cooper approached Camp and spoke to him, with the purpose of quelling the noise. As he turned away Cooper saw a glass flying towards him and instinctively put up a hand to protect himself, falling to the ground as he did so. His right hand was badly cut. Cooper's wife at once called the police and an ambulance. It transpired that a tendon in Cooper's hand had been severed. Despite an operation there was a traumatic reaction to the injury, resulting in the partial loss of movement in the hand.

21. **John Blake**, an unemployed graduate of 31 and an habitual heavy drinker, was very drunk when he was assaulted in a pub. He couldn't remember the attack in any detail, but several regulars in the pub where the incident occurred were afterwards able to tell him something of what had happened. Apparently Blake became involved in an argument with a stranger concerning whose turn it was at the pool table. Some ten minutes later this person approached Blake and felled him with a couple of punches. When Blake came to he staggered from the pub before realising that his ankle was badly damaged. He asked a passer-by to call an ambulance. It transpired that Blake, whose face was badly bruised, had also somehow broken an ankle. The fracture required pinning and Blake was in plaster for six weeks.

22. **Helen Evans** lives with her boyfriend in his house in the St Paul's district of Bristol. She had experienced several attacks from this partner previously. On this occasion Evans, who is alcoholic, had returned from one of her periodic lone drinking bouts when she and her boyfriend began a violent argument. Evans has little recollection of the incident but believes that she began throwing things about, as she has done in the past, whereupon her boyfriend struck her on the ear. She has confused memories of running from the house and spending the night at the home of a woman friend. Her boyfriend sought her out there the next day and they agreed to resume their relationship. Because Evans was bleeding from the ear she went to the hospital where she was kept in for observation and a possible brain-scan.

23. **Robin Smailes**, aged 33, was stabbed in the back by his wife. The couple have been married for 13 years and have two sons. The stabbing was the culmination of an argument which arose after Smailes discovered that his wife had been out socialising rather than at work, as she had claimed. In the face of Smailes' fury at this deception which, he feared, concealed marital infidelity, Mrs Smailes seized a knife from the draining board and stabbed her husband, possibly damaging his kidneys. Smailes spent several days in hospital.

24. **Paul Dunne** was the victim of an attack by his girlfriend's former boyfriend, a serving Royal Marine. He suffered damage to his jaw and the loss of several teeth. The assault, which was witnessed by

Dunne's girlfriend, took place in a club after a chance meeting and was immediately reported to the police by the couple.

25. **Edward Jones** was a passenger in his girlfriend's car when another car cut in front of them, preventing them from making a left-hand turn. The drivers exchanged V signs. Then, as Jones' girlfriend was once more manoeuvring to make the turn, the driver of the second car, Peter White, drew up beside them, got out of his car and approached the front passenger door. Jones also got out and words were exchanged between the two men. White pushed Jones backwards and then, as Jones came towards him, let fly a blow which caught Jones on the side of the chin, breaking his jaw. White immediately returned to his car and drove off, but not before Jones' girlfriend had noted the car registration number.

26. **William Straker** was jumped on from behind, knocked to the ground and kicked by an unseen attacker. Straker, who had been out drinking with friends one night to celebrate his birthday, was listening to his personal stereo as he walked home. He was knocked unconscious in the attack and only came round in hospital where he spent several nights, recovering from severe cuts to his face, a fractured cheekbone and bruising to his ribs and shoulders.

27. **Kevin Pilcher**, aged 22, has himself been imprisoned for assault. On this occasion he was attacked outside one of the most favoured (and most volatile) drinking places for young people in Bristol. Pilcher got into an argument with another youth in the pub – someone who, it transpired, was the brother of one of the pub bouncers. When Pilcher and his friends left the pub this bouncer and some of his cohorts followed them. Pilcher's friends fled the scene as he was set upon by several bouncers. Pilcher was given a severe beating, his most serious injury being a fractured cheekbone which necessitated several days' hospital treatment.

28. **Ronald Pratt** is a probationer police constable. While on night-shift he and a colleague were called to a disturbance in which two men were said to be vandalising a bus. The officers followed a trail of blood which led them to the Accident and Emergency Department of the Bristol Royal Infirmary. As they arrived two men matching the descriptions which they had been given emerged from the hospital. The men were questioned and the officers moved to

arrest them. As Pratt glanced down to retrieve his handcuffs he was struck full in the face by a powerful blow from one of the suspects. The blow knocked him unconscious. His assailant ran off, pursued by Pratt's colleague. The other man remained to help Pratt and in due course assisted him into the hospital. Pratt's nose was broken and the surrounding cartilege damaged. He needed a second operation to resolve breathing problems.

29. **Ranjit Patel** was hit in the face by Jim Sanderson, with whom he was in dispute over building repair work. Patel felt it necessary to recall Sanderson to finish some plastering which he considered had not been properly completed. He refused payment until the work was done. Sanderson agreed to improve the plastering but when he finished and called Patel to look at the result, Patel was still dissatisfied and unwilling to pay. Words were exchanged and then, according to Patel, Sanderson unleashed a single blow of great force, catching him on the side of the face. As Sanderson made to leave, Patel told him that he was going to phone the police 'because you have done a wrong'. Sanderson also phoned the police soon after the incident, apparently to put his side of the story. Patel suffered facial bruising as well as damage to his nose and cheekbone. This had to be repaired under general anaesthetic.

30. **Nigel Jenks**, aged 23, was assaulted late one Friday night in the city centre. He and a group of friends had been in a club when the place erupted in a series of fights. Jenks was walking to a taxi-rank when a girl started shouting at him, accusing him of having punched her boyfriend. The next thing Jenks recalls is recovering consciousness in hospital. Apparently someone had run up behind him and delivered a severe blow to the side of his head, possibly with a brick. Jenks suffered a hairline fracture of his right cheekbone, a badly swollen right eye, and an assortment of cuts and bruises.

31. **Gerald Abbott**, a retired police officer of 59, was attacked by a youth in the street. He was punched in the face, knocked to the ground and then kicked. The assault left him with a slashed upper lip, cuts and grazes around the upper part of his face, and facial bruising. The attack happened as Abbott was passing a group of teenagers late one evening. He noticed an argument going on between two members of the group – a young man and a girl – and appears to have offered some comment. This provoked the young

man into attacking him. When he recovered consciousness Abbott found his attacker had disappeared, though several of the youths in the group stayed to call an ambulance.

32. **Walter Drobny**, a Polish veteran of World War II who is now aged 76, suffered head injuries in a robbery. He was putting his car away in the garages below the flats where he lives when he noticed some youths standing in the shadows. As he was closing the garage door he felt a heavy blow to the back of his neck and fell forward on to the concrete surface. Drobny's attackers grabbed his wallet and ran off. Drobny was able to stagger back to his flat. A neighbour telephoned the police while Drobny went with his wife to hospital.

33. **Anthony Niblett**, a social worker, was the victim of an attack which took place in the street but originated in a gay club. Niblett had in the past received threats from his attacker, Ian Mather, because of his friendship with Mather's partner. On the evening of the attack Niblett was drinking with friends when he noticed an argument going on between Mather and Mather's partner, culminating in the throwing of a glass. It appears that Niblett then caught Mather's attention, following which a glass was thrown at *him*. Niblett claims to have ignored this, although he did subsequently exchange some words with Mather's partner. Soon afterwards Niblett and his friends left the club, closely followed by Mather. As Mather was getting into a taxi Niblett shouted some obscenity at him. At this Mather approached Niblett and struck him hard in the face, knocking him to the ground, and then kicked him where he lay. One of Niblett's companions called the police who arrived promptly, although not before Mather had left the scene.

34. **Linda Hutt**, aged 37, lives alone in a council flat. She has a 12-year-old daughter who lives with Hutt's parents. Hutt and the child's father have not lived together since shortly after the birth of their child, although he still visits her, sometimes staying for days at a time. Hutt has suffered repeated injury from this man. She says it is a result of his 'moodiness'. On this occasion the couple were arguing and Hutt made as if to leave the room. At this her boyfriend flung a glass at her, cutting her hand badly. Hutt asked her boyfriend to drive her to hospital but he refused. She set off on foot but then, thinking the journey would be too much for her, returned home and managed to persuade him to drive her. He dropped her at

the hospital door and disappeared. Hutt suffered tendon damage to her hand.

35. **Matthew Collins**, while out for a drink with his girlfriend, came face to face with an acquaintance, Steven Patten. The two young men had been at school together and were mutually antipathetic. On this occasion a few insults were traded before Patten, who is considerably more powerfully built than Collins, launched a rugby tackle at him, causing Collins to fall backwards through a shop window with Patten on top of him. Both youths were cut and, bleeding profusely, sought assistance in the adjacent pub. With them went Collins' girlfriend and four or five of Patten's companions who had apparently witnessed the incident. The landlord called the police. A tendon in Collins' hand was severed, causing long-term damage.

36. **Sandra Hind** was out for an evening with some female friends in the city centre when she was assaulted. The club in which Hind and her friends had spent the evening was due to close and Hind went out into the street slightly ahead of her companions. When they joined her Hind saw that one of them was involved in a heated argument with another girl, a stranger. This girl had apparently accused Hind's friend of attempting to steal her handbag. The two girls were locked in a noisy altercation when a man intervened, threatening Hind's friend. At this Hind herself joined in, challenging the man who promptly grabbed her by the arm and kicked her in the leg. This caused Hind to fall through the shop window behind her, cutting and scarring her chest. Her assailant immediately ran off.

37. **Jessie Roberts** is aged 34, has three children, and is a professional shoplifter. Her boyfriend, a trainee social worker, assaults her regularly. This time she had been subjected to a sustained beating, the bruises on her back and shoulders being clearly visible at the time of interview. Following the attack Jessie rang the police, who came to the house at 3 a.m. The boyfriend answered the door. The officers did not enter the premises but asked to see Jessie. She showed herself from a first-floor window but, with her boyfriend standing behind her, she said nothing and the police left.

38. **Brian Miller**, aged 23, was injured late one evening in a street attack. He and his brother-in-law were waiting to catch a bus home

after an evening's pub crawl. They were both attacked, possibly with a metal bar, and knocked unconscious. Neither man saw his attacker(s). An ambulance was summoned by a passing police car. Each brother suffered a broken nose, along with cuts and bruises. Brian Miller also suffered some damage to his shoulder.

39. **John Enwright**, having taken early retirement from the police force, now works as a warehouse clerk at a weighbridge. He told us that he arrived at work at 6.30 a.m. one January morning and began his usual routine of taking the day's money from the safe in the yard office. At this point he had to go to the toilet, leaving the money on the counter in his office. When he returned to the office Enwright noticed that the safe door was not properly closed; as he stepped forward to shut it he was struck on the head. He was knocked unconscious and only came fully to his senses when he reached hospital. The weapon used was half a breeze block. The investigating police officers formed the view that Enwright himself was the robber and that he had inflicted the injury upon himself as a cover for the robbery.

40. **Patrick Mates** was beaten up with a snooker cue in a Bristol pub. His assailant was known to him, being his cousin's husband. Apparently this man, who was already subject to a suspended prison sentence for assault, 'went berserk'. The police were called but Mates informed them that, given the family relationship, he did not wish to press charges.

41. **Dave Knowles** is an epileptic and a heavy drinker who has suffered considerable victimisation in the past. He works as a newspaper seller and lives in St Paul's under conditions of severe deprivation. Knowles gave us a confused account of this particular assault, the details of which remain obscure. He told us that he was walking home late one night carrying his day's takings, amounting to over £100, in his newspaper sack. As he walked down a narrow alleyway near his flat Knowles was jumped on by two men, who threatened him with a knife; he struggled and was slashed on the arm and neck before the men ran off with the money. Knowles made his way home and his girlfriend then went out to phone for an ambulance. He received 14 stitches to the cut on his arm. (An alternative source of Knowles' injuries may have been his girlfriend, a formidable young woman with whom he has a stormy relationship.)

42. **Anthony Glover**, a recent school-leaver, had spent the day at a football match before visiting several pubs and finally going to a party in a town a few miles from his home village. Having been turned away from the party, Glover and a male friend went to a recreation ground to wait for a lift home. Some local youngsters were hanging around there and, according to Glover, he and his friend were approached by three youths who accused them of having been involved in a recent assault upon a local lad. A fight ensued in the course of which Glover was knocked to the ground and kicked. A blow to the head knocked him out and he only regained full consciousness in hospital. The attack left Glover with cuts and bruising to his head; his friend escaped more lightly with a black eye and bruised lips.

43. **William Kenny**, aged 31, was assaulted in the car park of a pub in Wells. Kenny, who had drunk several pints of beer, got into an argument with another customer who accused him of spitting on the floor. The other man, Bob Little, is a well-known local character who, according to both Kenny and the police, possesses formidable strength and physical presence. At the time Kenny did not recognise Little, but he subsequently realised that he had been attacked by him before. On this occasion Little followed Kenny to the toilet where he verbally abused him before forcing him out into the pub car park. There he struck Kenny over the head with a weapon – probably a brick. Kenny, who had a badly cut head, was brought to Bristol by ambulance.

44. **Royston Kilmore** is a 'dosser', probably in his forties. On the night he was attacked he was staying, as he frequently does, in a city centre night shelter. A fight broke out in the course of which Kilmore's nose was broken and his face badly bruised. It seems that Kilmore, who was very drunk at the time, was set upon by four men, also regulars at the shelter. Shelter staff broke up the fight and called the police.

45. **Jonathan Musgrove**, a police officer, was celebrating New Year's Eve with his wife in a local pub when he was the recipient of a single crashing blow to his jaw. According to Musgrove the accident resulted from his being 'in the wrong place at the wrong time'. His assailant, a local youth, had just had a violent disagreement with his girlfriend and as she left the pub, pushing past Musgrove, the youth

followed her and lashed out at random. The blow knocked Musgrove to the floor but he was able to get up swiftly and pursue the young man, catching up with him just outside the pub. There then followed an angry exchange in the course of which Musgrove identified himself as an off-duty police officer and secured the name of his attacker, who then left. Musgrove suffered a hairline fracture of the jaw and the loss of several teeth.

46. **Peter Barton** and the two friends with whom he had, as usual, spent Friday night in the local pubs, were accosted in the street near his home. Two strangers attacked one of Barton's friends with fists and heels, karate-style. Barton attempted to intervene and was himself set upon. Both his friends ran away. After a few minutes the attackers themselves made off and Barton was able to make his way home. Barton and his friend received similar injuries: a black eye, cut lip, bruises and loosened teeth. While being treated for these in the Accident and Emergency Department later that night the two men told their story to a police officer whom they happened to encounter.

47. **Bill Ray**, a single man of 28, told us that he was attacked in the street as he got off a bus on his way to work. At the time of the incident Ray was working as a barman and the assault took place in the early evening. Ray was hit from behind, possibly with a heavy bar of some kind. He fell to the ground and was further hit in the face and kicked in the stomach and legs. He said that he caught no more than a glimpse of his attackers, whom he could describe only as two white youths. Despite his injuries Ray managed to make his way home by bus but on the following day his legs were so stiff and bruised that he sought hospital treatment.

48. **Jonathan Dowson** is a 'biker', currently unemployed. He was assaulted while drinking with a friends in a city centre pub one lunch-time. During a game of pool with an acquaintance, also a biker, an argument developed and the two went outside to settle it (verbally, according to Dowson). Thinking that the matter was closed Dowson turned to go back inside, whereupon he was struck on the back of the head with a pool cue. The blow caused a deep cut to his scalp and the shock of the assault precipitated an asthma attack. Dowson's companions called an ambulance. He received six stitches to the cut.

49. **Matthew Howell** was assaulted in St Paul's, near the bail hostel where he has lived since his release from prison. He was just round the corner from the hostel when a man approached and asked him for a light. As Howell complied, he was offered drugs for sale. He refused them and walked on. A few seconds later he received a crashing blow to the back of his head. Howell's pockets were rifled and the £5 which he had on him was removed before his assailant ran off.

50. **Steven Godden** is a businessman aged 39. He told us that he was in Bristol on business when he became lost in the St Paul's area while looking for a short cut to the motorway. As he was making a three-point turn his driver's door was opened by a man who began hitting him and demanding money. A second man forced his way into the seat beside Godden and, threatening him with a knife, started rifling the car. (Apart from a watch and pen he found little of value, since Godden's wallet, containing a substantial sum of money, was in his inside pocket; Godden's lap-top computer lay on the back seat but was apparently not noticed by the robbers.) Godden put up a struggle, eventually managing to force his way out of the car. As he did this his left trouser-leg was slashed from top to bottom. Once out of the car Godden banged on the roof of the car in an attempt to attract attention. He saw a police van on the motorway; his attackers may also have spotted it, for at this point they made off. The police van arrived shortly afterwards.

51. **Josephine Macdonald** is a young Belfast woman of middle-class background who told us that she had for some time 'dropped out' and lived as a traveller. At the time of the assault she was living in St Paul's and working as a clerk for the city council. Macdonald was attacked by an ex-boyfriend, Jeremy Allen, when she went to visit a man with whom she had recently begun a relationship. This man lived on a boat in the city dock and it was dark by the time Macdonald arrived. She found her friend was not at home and was about to climb into the boat to wait for him when Allen approached, warning her to keep away from her new friend. Then, as Macdonald began to speak to him, he hit her in the face. Macdonald was knocked to the ground and kicked as she lay there. She screamed in an effort to attract attention but no one intervened. Allen disappeared and Macdonald, who was bleeding from cuts to her head and had lost her glasses, sought help in a nearby pub.

52. **Julian Davies**, a man in his thirties, was the victim of a street attack in the St Paul's area where he lives. Davies went out at about 9 o'clock one night to buy some cigarettes. A man approached him and asked him for a light. Almost immediately Davies felt himself pushed up against a wall and he was then hit, possibly by a second man. He can remember no other details of the incident, which left him bruised and mildly concussed. He believed that his pockets had been rifled but afterwards he found nothing missing. Later that evening he sought hospital treatment.

53. **Amanda Britton** and the man with whom she had been living for seven months were engaged in a heated discussion about the Gulf War. Both had been drinking. Suddenly the boyfriend grabbed Britton and flung her across the room. She hit her head on a door, breaking her nose. Britton attempted to retaliate, but was then clawed in the face and punched in the eye. She ran from the flat and was picked up by a passing police car and given a lift to the home of a friend.

54. **Steve Tufnell**, aged 20, told us that he was enjoying an evening out in a city pub in a foursome including his sister, when a stranger who was drinking at the next table reached over and took a cigarette from Tufnell's sister. Tufnell remonstrated with him, whereupon he was hit hard in the face, the blow breaking his nose and knocking him unconscious. Tufnell can remember nothing more of the attack, but has been told by friends that as he lay on the floor he was kicked by his original assailant and two other youths.

55. **Donald Burke** was attacked late at night as he was waiting with his wife in the Accident and Emergency Department of the Bristol Royal Infirmary, he having accompanied her there when she sought treatment for a cut arm. Also in the waiting area was a young man, Bill Winter. He was heavily intoxicated and had been taken to the hospital by the police, apparently having been injured in the course of a fight in the city centre. When Burke went to the lavatory Winter followed him. No words were exchanged but Winter head-butted Mr Burke, breaking his nose and knocking him to the floor. He then ran off but was picked up shortly afterwards by the police not far from the hospital.

56. **Nick Castle** is a young trainee baker who had recently moved to Bristol and found temporary work in one of the most volatile city centre pubs. Late on Christmas Eve, when the place was especially noisy and crowded and the atmosphere more than usually combustible, Castle was going about his job collecting empties from the tables when he was punched in the face by a customer and his nose broken. By his own account, he had simply asked a group of drinkers to pick up their glasses while he removed the empties. The attack took Castle entirely by surprise. He fell to the ground and was almost immediately manhandled by a bouncer. The manageress then appeared and ordered Castle to the kitchen. A furious altercation ensued between the manageress and Castle, who ended the affair by giving his notice and walking out.

57. **Edward Billingston** was leaving a club in the city centre after a night out with friends when he was punched in the face by a total stranger. A man had pushed in front of Billingston while the two of them were collecting their coats from the club cloakroom. Billingston had objected to being pushed aside and been met by a stream of invective. As he left the club he was hit. He assumed that his assailant was the man he had encountered in the cloakroom but the attack was so sudden that he did not see his assailant. Billingston was knocked to the ground and his nose broken. There were no witnesses.

58. **Paul Warren** and two fellow university students were attacked in the street as they, plus the 16-year-old brother of one of them, were walking to a nightclub. Warren and his friends had been conscious of being followed by two men for a little while. As they neared the city centre and entered a subway they looked behind, to discover that the two men had become ten. Before they could run the students were set upon and knocked to the ground. They were then kicked in the face and body. One of them handed over his wallet containing about £25. This didn't stem the flow of violence immediately, though after a little while the attackers ran off. Meanwhile the younger brother had managed to get away. He ran into the street where one of the gang confronted him, demanding money. He too surrendered his wallet. The students reported the incident to the police the following day.

59. **Annie Cresswell** was attacked on New Year's Eve by her partner, Patrick Mason. Two weeks before this attack she had received out-patient treatment for facial bruising inflicted by Mason. Cresswell, who had herself been drinking, was in the house with Brendan, aged 7, the youngest of her seven surviving children; Mason was out drinking with friends. When he returned a row developed; Mason began hitting Cresswell and, she alleges, threatened her with a knife. Brendan ran next door and from there telephoned the police.

60. **Sally Chapman** was attacked by her mother's common-law husband, Michael Dwyer. Although she was brought up in care and later fostered, Chapman keeps in touch with her mother and now lives close to her in St Paul's. The mother is alcoholic, as is the mother's boyfriend. Chapman alleges that Dwyer has been violent towards her mother for some years. One evening Chapman went round to the rooms occupied by her mother and Dwyer and, possibly emboldened by drink, began abusing Dwyer verbally. He in turn punched her, bruising her face and, according to Chapman, threatening her with a knife and a hammer. The mother and the landlord eventually intervened and Chapman left. After seeking hospital treatment Chapman reported the assault to the police.

61. **Alice Smythe**, aged 39 and the mother of two children, was punched in the face during a row with her boyfriend, Daniel Biggs who, according to Smythe, is alcoholic. The couple had been out drinking when an initially low-key argument exploded. Smythe made a couple of provocative remarks to Biggs, who responded by striking her full in the face, causing her to bleed from the nose and mouth. Biggs at once called an ambulance.

62. **Sean Bradenham**, a university student, was working as a security guard at a student ball when he confronted a man apparently queue-jumping and attempting to obtain a champagne breakfast to which he was not entitled. An initial verbal exchange was followed, some ten minutes later, by a further confrontation in which Bradenham, while trying to manhandle the trouble-maker to the back of the queue, was first grabbed by the lapels and then head-butted. Bradenham tried to retaliate but a friend of the assailant pulled him off. The assailant and his friend were evicted from the ball by other security guards. Bradenham's nose was broken.

63. **Robert James**, a university student, was on his way home late one evening in the company of three friends. As they were walking down a quiet back street they saw a noisy party of young men approaching them on the opposite side of the road. When the two groups drew level James and his friends came under a hail of objects, including bricks and bottles. They turned and ran, pursued by their attackers. James was grabbed from behind and laid into by four or five youths, who punched and head-butted him. James' friends ran off, as did James himself as soon as he was able to break away. His head was badly bruised and one eye blackened in the assault.

64. **David Elliston**, aged 26, was the victim of a 'bolt from the blue' assault perpetrated late one evening as he was on his way home from the pub. He had been drinking in the city centre with a group of friends and had consumed at least six pints of beer. After leaving the pub to catch a bus, Elliston passed a group of five or six young men, one of whom said something to him. Feeling threatened, Elliston said nothing and walked on. He then heard running footsteps behind him, turned, and had his legs kicked from under him. He was kicked again in the chest and believes that he blacked out briefly. When he came to a woman passer-by was trying to assist him; the group of youths was to be seen walking off down the road.

65. **Alison Browne**, who is alcoholic, lives with her husband and 27-year-old younger son. On this occasion she was, by her own account, drunk and argumentative when her son, infuriated by his mother's condition, kicked her about the legs and back. There had been other such attacks in the past. The next day there were further arguments and this led Mrs Browne to tell the manager of her local off-licence of the assault she had suffered the day before. The manager called the police.

66. **Rowena Macintosh**, a university postgraduate student, was attacked one evening as she was walking home through the city centre with her boyfriend. The couple were crossing the road when they had to move swiftly to avoid being hit by a car which was being driven, Macintosh considered, at reckless speed. Macintosh shouted and made a V sign at the driver who promptly drew up, got out of the car and confronted her. During a heated exchange Macintosh was verbally abused and pushed. The violence then escalated as the driver hit Macintosh on the side of the face. Punches were also

exchanged with the boyfriend, who proved no match for his antagonist. Macintosh suffered further blows, including one to the eye. Bystanders declined to intervene despite Rowena's urgings. After a time the driver took his leave and Macintosh's boyfriend summoned the police.

67. **Ann Parkinson**, a divorced woman of 40, was injured when a fight broke out in the house which she shares with two other women. Parkinson, a clerk working for the police, had returned from a night-shift and was trying to sleep when she was disturbed by the noise of drilling in another bedroom. On going down to the kitchen Parkinson was confronted by one of her fellow tenants, Patsy Cole, and Patsy's mother. (The person doing the drilling was Patsy's father.) After some argument Parkinson went back to bed, but when the noise continued she returned to the kitchen. There a quarrel broke out between the three women, developing into a physical skirmish in which, Parkinson alleges, she was slapped in the face and roughly handled by Patsy and her mother. Parkinson thrust Patsy's mother against the door. The mother's screams alerted her husband who burst into the kitchen, grabbed Parkinson by the head and kneed her several times before throwing her to the floor. The third tenant had been in her room throughout but did not intervene. The Coles then alerted the landlady who came round at once and, seeing Parkinson's battered and bruised condition, immediately evicted Mr and Mrs Cole from the house and gave Patsy notice to quit. Parkinson reported the incident to the police.

68. **Jane Bond** became embroiled in a fight with her boyfriend as a result of which she was bruised and cut on her face, neck and back. The couple were both very drunk when the outburst occurred. It was Bond who, by her own admission, struck the first blows. She explained this as a furious reaction to her boyfriend's regular heavy drinking, something which had led her to wish to end the relationship. Having been worsted by her boyfriend Bond broke free and ran from the flat to telephone the police.

69. **Louise Duke**, a student nurse, was walking with a group of girlfriends down a main street near the hospital late one night. A young man, Francis Melotti, passed them going in the opposite direction and as he did so he dropped a stick (possibly a builder's ruler). Duke picked this up and was carrying it when her companions noticed

that the man had turned and was following them down the road. Duke turned round to hand back the stick to its owner, who appeared to be smiling. In that instant he struck her hard across the face with the stick. When one of Duke's friends remonstrated with the stranger he struck her also. One of the girls flagged down a passing police car. Duke and her friend were taken for a tour of the vicinity in the hope that they might identify their assailant. They spotted him almost immediately and he was arrested after a violent struggle in which two police officers were injured.

70. **Darren Chandler** is a young man of 24 who has suffered repeated victimisation, partly no doubt because he is severely alcoholic and can himself be aggressive. This particular incident took place not far from Chandler's home on a desolate housing estate. Chandler, whose speech when interviewed was generally incoherent and his manner volatile, was vague about the details of the incident but said that he was attacked in the street by two youths aged about 15 or 16. His face was bruised and scratched. Someone from a nearby fish and chip shop called an ambulance.

71. **David Thompson** and his friend Michael Dobson were sitting outside the Accident and Emergency Department, having a smoke. Dobson had cut himself when falling on the dance floor of a club during a night out and was awaiting treatment, but a disturbance in the hospital had driven the men outside. As they were sitting on a ledge close to the hospital entrance a group of people emerged, one of whom was lashing out, shouting and swearing. This man, subsequently identified as Philip Cleese, approached Thompson and Dobson, said something inaudible and then struck out at Dobson, causing him momentarily to lose consciousness. As Thompson looked towards Dobson he too was struck and knocked backwards against the wall. At this point a police car appeared, the police having been called to deal with the disturbance inside the hospital.

72. **June Fell**, a divorcee in her sixties, was assaulted when she attempted to intervene in one of the habitual violent confrontations between her daughter Samantha Rice and Rice's boyfriend, Nick Somers. (Rice has two children by her estranged husband and a baby by Somers.) Fell was called to her daughter's house by her 11-year-old grandson, Rice's eldest child, who told her that a violent quarrel was taking place. When Fell arrived a few minutes later she found

the couple in the living room, Somers holding the baby. Fell told Somers that she intended to 'take out a summons' against him for hitting her grandchild. At this Somers put down the baby and advanced on Fell, catching her roughly by the throat. Fell dropped to the floor before getting to her feet and going to the house next door where a neighbour called the police.

73. **Melanie Morton**, who left home in her early teens and is now 18, lives in the home of a professional shoplifter Jessie Roberts (see case 37), and moves in a circle of petty criminals. Melanie had had a brief relationship with a young black man which she had decided to end. She then went to a pub which she had been in the habit of frequenting with this boyfriend, and got very drunk. As she was talking to another man her ex-boyfriend (of one day) punched her in the face. After Melanie left the pub he followed her and subjected her to repeated punches and kicks. Her assailant was restrained by onlookers. Melanie reported the assault to the police.

74. **John Wheaton** was attacked in circumstances which remain obscure. An unemployed man of 51, Wheaton lives in a dilapidated high-rise block on the outskirts of Bristol. He and his wife are both heavy drinkers and probably spend some of their time drinking on the streets in the city centre. Wheaton recounted a confused tale of many assaults in which he had apparently been variously victim and aggressor. This particular assault appears to have been perpetrated by two people, one of them a woman who, Wheaton claimed, had previously been involved in an attack on Wheaton's wife. What prompted the attack is not clear but Wheaton was apparently knocked to the ground and kicked. He took himself to hospital immediately afterwards.

75. **Alexander Thomas**, aged 33, was walking home in the company of two friends with whom he had celebrated Burns Night. They passed a youth in the act of climbing a wall and, it appeared, vandalising a dentist's signboard. Thomas called out 'Pack it in!'. The youth dropped off the wall, apparently deterred. Thomas made some further remark and continued walking, only to be jostled from behind by the youth who then hit him once in the mouth and again in the eye. The second blow knocked Thomas to the ground. At this point one of his companions began to scream, which brought three youths, friends of Thomas's attacker, back to the scene. The

incident resolved itself when the four youths walked off, having accepted the advice of Thomas's friend to 'cool it'.

76. **Lindy Stone**, 20, was taken to the police by her father after she had been punched in the face by her boyfriend, James Vaughan. Vaughan is the father of Stone's eight-month-old daughter. The relationship was marked by a history of violence and the particular assault which prompted Stone's father to take his daughter to the police was not the most serious that had occurred. On this occasion Vaughan, who had been out drinking over Christmas, returned drunk and aggressive on Boxing Day and went for Stone when she remonstrated with him about his absence.

77. **Julie Appleford**, a single woman of 32, was punched in the face during an argument with her brother. The argument, which took place in the house shared by Julie and her father, arose out of ill-feeling which had developed when the brother's wife and children had sought refuge with Julie and her father. The brother had a history of violent behaviour and threatened to harm Appleford further if she reported the incident to the police.

78. **Phil Deacon**, a young man of 25 who works as a shelf-filler in a supermarket, was attacked as he was on his way home from working a late shift. A group of about five youths, probably schoolchildren, approached Deacon as he stood at the bus-stop. One of the youths asked Deacon if he had any money and when he replied that he had none, forced a hand into Deacon's jacket pocket, where he had a personal stereo. Deacon managed to pull his assailant's hand away but was immediately punched hard in the chest. The youths walked off, leaving Deacon shocked and bruised. He at once reported the incident at the nearby police station.

79. **Robert Green**, a single man in his late twenties, went out with two friends one November evening to pick up a take-away meal from a cafe near his tower-block flat. Inside the cafe he and his friends encountered hostility from a group of six skinheads. This gang followed Green and his friends into the street and it soon became apparent to Green that there was going to be some kind of confrontation. In an attempt to avoid this the three men made a run for it, becoming separated in the process. Green returned to his flat alone but decided to go out again in order to search for his companions.

Almost immediately he came face to face with the skinheads. He tried to talk his way out of the situation but one of the group flung a plastic milk crate at him, hitting the side of his face. He once more took to his heels and was able to run back into the block of flats. Several days later Green sought hospital treatment for a deep cut on his cheekbone; he also reported the incident at his local police station.

80. **Paul White**, an ambulanceman, was attacked while on duty one night after answering a call to pick up a young man who had reportedly attempted suicide. The ambulance crew found the youth, bleeding from cut wrists, being held by two club bouncers who had come to his assistance in the street. Two plain clothes police officers, summoned by Ambulance Control, were watching the incident at a distance. White approached the youth and before he had a chance to speak was struck full in the face by a blow which felled him. His assailant attempted to hit him again but was restrained by the bouncers before being arrested, after some struggle, by the police officers. White suffered painful bruising to his neck and shoulder but was able to carry on with his shift.

81. **John Westcott**, aged 22, was injured in a pub fight. Westcott was out drinking with two friends late one Friday night. The pub, as was usual for that time, was extremely crowded and noisy. Westcott saw a stranger punch one of his friends in the face, apparently unprovoked, although Westcott subsequently discovered that this blow was precipitated by racial taunts. The blow knocked his friend unconscious. Westcott retaliated by striking the original assailant several times in the face before he himself was attacked by five or six other young men, at least one of whom was using a bottle as a weapon. Westcott's second friend joined in the mêlée, receiving a cut lip for his pains. Westcott's nose was broken and his face cut. Bouncers broke up the fight before police arrived.

82. **Kevin Grimsby** suffered a gash to his head in the course of a brawl outside a pub in his home village. Grimsby, a single man in his twenties, was drinking with three friends. The group decided to move on to a second pub and as they were entering the premises by a door from a dark alleyway Grimsby stopped to talk to someone whom he knew. In that instant, he says, he was hit on the side of the head. Grimsby hit back, leading to a free-for-all. Grimsby was kicked, punched and hit with a beer glass; one of his friends was

knocked unconscious. The fight was broken up by Grimsby's cousin, an off-duty police officer.

83. **Michael Elmes**, a student aged 19, was celebrating his younger brother Tim's eighteenth birthday in a city centre club with a small group of friends. Michael, who had consumed about six pints of beer during the evening, was on the dance floor when he noticed that a gang of four or five youths had forced their way onto the floor and were deliberately jostling the dancers. One of these youths collided heavily with Michael, knocking him to the floor. At this point Tim intervened to protect Michael and both brothers were then punched by several of the youths. At the approach of a bouncer the attackers made off and the Elmes party were themselves escorted from the premises.

84. **Daniel Batstone**, who is strikingly punk in appearance, was dancing on a crowded floor in a city centre club when he was jostled from behind. Batstone resisted the jostling whereupon he was at once punched fiercely and repeatedly in the ribs by three or four assailants. Batstone, who is strongly built, hit back several times before pushing his way straight to the nearest exit.

85. **Bob Deane**, who is in his sixties and approaching retirement, works as one of the head porters in Bristol University Student Union. He was on duty one Friday night when trouble developed in a bar on the second floor. On investigating he found that two young people, a man and a woman, both very drunk, were behaving offensively to other customers in the bar, shouting obscenities and attempting to grab people. As the bar manager escorted the woman out of the bar Deane and a fellow porter took hold of the man in order to propel him down the stairs and out of the building. On reaching the ground floor, Deane's attention was distracted for a moment and his captive managed to break free. In doing so he pushed Deane backwards against a drinks vending machine. As a result of the incident Deane suffered long-term damage to his shoulder.

86. **Patsy McShea** is a residential social worker in a children's home. She suffered a broken bone in her hand when attempting to break up a fight between two girls. One of the girls turned on McShea and in the course of a tussle kicked her right hand.

87.   Mushtak Iqbal owns a thriving general store. He was punched once in the chest by a much younger white man who lives in a guest-house opposite the shop. There had been several disagreements between the two men in the past. On this occasion Iqbal's adversary accused him of having insulted his girlfriend. Iqbal called the police after the incident and also went to hospital. Hospital staff found no significant injury but Iqbal says he suffered chest pain for two weeks.

88.   Sally Chapman (see also case 60) told us that she was 'glassed' by a stranger while in a gay club. Chapman was drinking at a table with a deaf and dumb friend when another drinker began insulting her. She was provoked into shouting a retort, whereupon a glass was flung at her. The glass broke over her head, cutting her scalp slightly. Her assailant ran from the club, pursued by the club manager.

89.   Darren Strudwick, aged 27, was injured in a pub brawl. He told us that he had intervened in a confrontation between a youth and two bouncers and had as a result been seized by the bouncers, who rammed his head against a mirror, causing a cut above his eye. According to Strudwick he had decided to intervene initially because the odds against the youth were unfair. The bouncers ejected Strudwick from the pub, the youth having made off. Bar staff called the police, who found Strudwick outside the pub and put him into their car, apparently with the intention of charging him. On enquiring in the pub, however, they were told that the manager didn't want the matter pursued.

90.   Alan Small, a university student, had been drinking for some six hours or more in celebration of the completion of his final exams when he became involved in a violent incident, the details of which remain obscure. Small was standing at a bar in the company of a friend, Peter Wilkins, also drunk, and two acquaintances, younger students who had drunk very little. It appears that Small got into an argument with a stranger and was struck in the face. Wilkins intervened, the violence escalated and a number of other customers joined in. The two younger students eventually managed to extricate Small and Wilkins, while bar staff called the police. As Small left the premises he wiped his bloodied hand across the face of a customer standing near the door, one Patrick Tapnell, leading to further argument but (so Tapnell assured us) no further violence.

91. **Donald Cruikshank**, a young man with a history of petty offences, snatched a handbag from the back of a parked car. As he was running away, an unmarked police car, on surveillance in the area, gave chase towards the city centre. A passer-by joined in the pursuit and he and the driver of the police car eventually caught up with the fugitive on a footbridge where there was a tussle during which the police officer was bitten on his forearm. Cruikshank was arrested and taken by car to the police station. He subsequently claimed that he had been deliberately knocked down by the police car as he ran along the pavement and then, following his arrest, had been roughed up in the back of the police car. At Cruikshank's request he was seen by a police doctor and, when released from police custody, was treated in hospital for minor cuts and bruises.

92. **Mike Webber**, a university student, was injured in a street fight. He was walking back to his hostel late one night with four friends, after a pub crawl, when his group passed four youths walking in the opposite direction. Hostile words were exchanged. A few minutes later Webber, as he stood waiting in the street for two of his companions to come out of a 'take-away', noticed that his other two friends had stayed behind and were apparently being invited to a fight by the youths whom the group had just encountered. Webber went back to 'help'. He pushed two of the youths into a shop doorway, one into a skip, and started to fight with the fourth. Webber, who was extremely drunk, was worsted in the struggle, during which his face was cut and bruised.

93. **Bill Winter**, a heavy drinker, could remember nothing of the assault which resulted in his being taken to the Accident and Emergency Department in a police car. Having recently parted from his girl-friend of three years, Winter had been drinking heavily for three days. He had that morning been fired by his father, for whom he worked as a painter and decorator. He spent the rest of the day drinking in the city centre and it was there that he was picked up by a police car and taken to hospital for treatment to a cut head. Winter described himself to hospital admission staff as the victim of an assault. He subsequently attacked Donald Burke in the hospital toilets (case 55).

Notes

1 INTRODUCTION

1 Social historians record that it was in the eighteenth century that criminal courts began to prosecute and punish violent conduct which would previously have been ignored (Beattie 1984).
2 We exclude all violence from which any element of intention is lacking, so we leave out of account all road accidents, no matter that one of the parties may be considered to have driven recklessly or dangerously. We also leave out of consideration violent incidents for which there is (arguably) corporate rather than individual responsibility, as in the case of 'accidents' at work. Nor, third, are we concerned with violence which is welcomed by the victim, as in sado-masochistic acts. We realise that some of the above distinctions are not necessarily clear-cut and that all raise issues of considerable importance within the criminal law (Clarkson and Keating 1994: 230ff), but they are nonetheless marginal to the issues we wish to explore in this book.
3 *The Times*, 24 March 1993; *Independent*, 25 March 1993.
4 Board of Visitors, HMP Wandsworth (1992), Annual Report: 5.
5 'Victims who fought back and won', *The Sunday Times*, 27 March 1994.
6 The Law Commission has proposed a new categorisation: Law Com. No. 218 (1993), Cmnd. 2370.
7 *Social Trends*, Table 12.2, Vol. 24, 1994.
8 *Ibid.*
9 Digest 2, *Information on the Criminal Justice System in England and Wales* (1993), Home Office, Research and Statistics Department, London: HMSO): 60.
10 Michael Jack: speech to The Howard League Annual Conference, 9 September 1992, New College, Oxford.
11 *Social Trends*, Vol. 22, 1992.
12 People who fall prey to violence are more likely to suffer multiple victimisation than are those who suffer property crimes. Many incidents of violence are perpetrated by drunken offenders. *The 1992 British Crime Survey*: 86. Home Office Research Study 132, Pat Mayhew *et al.* (1993). Home Office Research and Planning Unit Report. London: HMSO.
13 When assaults are categorised by their circumstances, the largest number comprise domestic assaults (estimated at 520,000 in 1991). *Ibid.*, p. 84.

14 'Muggings' and assaults in and around the home are most likely to be reported, the reporting rate being estimated at about 50 per cent. About a third of work-related, street and pub assaults are reported to the police. Offences involving strangers are, in general, much less likely to be reported. *Ibid.*, pp. 95, 96.

15 *Social Trends*, Vol. 24, 1994.

16 *Criminal Victimisation in the Industrialised World: key findings of the 1989 and 1992 International Crime Surveys*, J. Van Dijk and P. Mayhew. The Hague: Ministry of Justice, 1993.

17 *Ibid.*

18 *Social Trends*, Vol. 22: Introduction.

19 *The Guardian*, 29.10.92.

20 House of Commons (1993) Memorandum of Evidence to Home Affairs Select Committee on Domestic Violence, p. 25.

21 Sir Frederick Lawton, 'Leaving the law to the experts', *The Times*, 8 January 1991.

22 For an authoritative account of different degrees of intention in violent acts, see R.A. Duff (1990).

23 Attempting to grade assaults on a scale of seriousness is inevitably a difficult and controversial exercise. Clearly the criminal law hierarchy of seriousness (grievous bodily harm with intent; malicious wounding; actual bodily harm; battery and assault) was too crude to be of any utility. On the other hand surveys have been conducted on the general public (Sellin and Wolfgang 1964) and crime victims (Sparks *et al.* 1977) in which participants have been asked to rank offences in order of seriousness. In developing our own ranking we sought to reflect the harm caused and, at the same time, to view the assault as an event in context. So we were assessing both harm *and* culpability (Von Hirsch 1985), although we confined ourselves to aggravating or mitigating factors surrounding the particular incident. Thus while we took into account the location of the assault and the relationship between victim and assailant, we did not consider extraneous factors such as the prevalence of a particular category of assault or the offender's previous convictions.

The following factors were taken into consideration: (i) actual physical injury; (ii) potential for more serious injury or, conversely, a recognition that the severity of injury was in some part a matter of chance, or ill-fortune; (iii) degree of threat, taking into account the relative strengths of victim and attacker; (iv) use of a weapon; (v) emotional or psychological harm; (vi) duration of attack; and (vii) provocation by the victim. As a small validation exercise we asked twenty colleagues to rank the assaults drawn from different points on our seriousness scale. There was substantial agreement (although not quite unanimity) in respect of those assaults which figured in the top and bottom 25 per cent of our scale; there was considerable variation in the rank order assigned to those assaults which we (and our testers) placed in the middle range. We think that this is inevitable given the subjective nature of many of the criteria employed.

24 On this theme, see Gottfredson and Gottfredson 1989: vii.

2 THE REALITY OF ASSAULT

1 *Social Trends*, Vol. 22, 1992, Table 12.9.
2 This may be because African–Caribbeans and Asians are less likely to attend for hospital treatment, or perhaps they were less inclined to co-operate with our study.
3 All names given in this book are pseudonyms. The case number reflects the ranking which we assigned to each case on our scale of seriousness, 1 being the most serious and 93 being the most trivial. Brief outlines of each incident referred to in this book appear in Appendix B.
4 Police records of violent crime in 1984 showed that 21 per cent of serious woundings occurred in pubs, discos and other places of entertainment (Walmsley 1986: 62).
5 Although, as Levi points out, it cannot be said that drink is sufficient or even necessary for the commission of such offences (Levi 1994: 336).
6 Many attempts at classification of assault are in fact classifications of location. For example, Gottfredson (1984) (drawing on data from the 1982 British Crime Survey) indicated (Table A:3, p. 39) that 19 per cent of common assaults reported to and recorded by the police took place in pubs, discos, and places of entertainment, often at weekends, while domestic violence and assaults in the workplace each accounted for 12 per cent. In relation to the more serious offence of wounding, 21 per cent of offences occurred in pubs, discos and places of entertainment, while 24 per cent occurred in the home. These figures cannot be taken as an indication of the true level of violence in these different settings. Under-reporting and under-recording is a feature of *all* assault, but perhaps especially of that which takes place in a 'domestic' context. A Home Office study based on police returns suggested that 29 per cent of assaults were perpetrated in the street; 15 per cent were 'domestic'; 9 per cent occurred in pubs; and 6 per cent involved an attack on a public servant (Davidoff and Greenhorn 1991).
7 As indicated in Chapter 1, we deliberately exclude violence which lacks any element of intentionality, such as road traffic accidents, and likewise all forms of so-called 'corporate' violence. We are concerned with deliberate, unwelcome, interpersonal violence.

3 HARM AND REPORTING

1 Mayhew (1984) has observed that: 'Past victimisations often do not seem memorable enough to be recalled for survey interviewers, and even those which are remembered are frequently trivial and of little import; they are part of life's vicissitudes, not ineffectively coped with by victims with help from family, friends and insurance premiums.' See also Gottfredson, 1989: 212.
2 All had been visited by representatives of Victim Support Schemes: they are unlikely, therefore, to be a wholly representative sample.
3 An organisation for partners or relatives of problem drinkers.
4 Domestic homicides generally follow a history of violence.
5 The 1984 British Crime Survey reported that some 91 per cent of offences

known to the police had been brought to their attention by victims or their families (Hough and Mayhew 1985: 19).

6 This, it should be said, is more a feature of the US than the UK literature. Hough and Mayhew (1985: 21) observe that 'although reporting increases with seriousness, many crimes rated highly on the seriousness scale go unreported, and many low ratings are reported'.

4 THE VICTIM AND THE POLICE

1 Yarsuvat is explicitly referring to regimes under which the victim is granted the *right* to withdraw his or her complaint – in the UK the victim has no such right, but our point is that he or she does have this power in practice.
2 See Smith (1989) for an overview of research in this area. As far as the police are concerned the sobriquet 'domestic' seems to be applied to any violence arising from a private quarrel, but we confine use of this term to assaults upon a sexual and/or marital partner or ex-partner.
3 Which persists even after the considerable change of emphasis in police policies relating to domestic violence following from the Metropolitan Police initiatives and the Home Office circular 60/1990.
4 The police quite explicitly direct many women towards civil remedies.
5 Williams (1976), in her study based on data from a Prosecutor's Management Information System in the US Attorney's Office for the District of Columbia, concludes that judgments about the victim's likely impact in court will be most telling in relation to the initial decision to prosecute. Few victims are actually exposed to judge and jury – decisions about their value as witnesses ensure that this is so.
6 In the case of Purnell the police went to the lengths of offering her alternative accommodation – an offer which she declined.

5 THE POLICE AND THE DEMANDS OF THE LEGAL PROCESS

1 Police and Criminal Evidence Act 1984.
2 There are frequent press reports of witness intimidation. See for instance *The Sunday Times*, 3 April 1994, 'Trials collapse as fear silences witnesses', which refers to over 300 cases abandoned nationally as a result of suspected witness intimidation.

6 POLICE CASE CONSTRUCTION

1 Although, as we have sown, the police are prepared to admit what appears to be mitigating evidence.
2 For a fuller discussion of the significance of the fact that the police 'go first', see Roberts and Willmore (1993).

7 VICTIMS IN COURT

1   Michael Howard, Home Secretary, in a speech accepting the recommendations of the Royal Commission on Criminal Justice, 1993, reported in *The
Daily Telegraph*, 27 November 1993.
2   The wording of the Code for Crown Prosecutors, para 6.7, suggests that the
victim interest is not identical with the public interest but should be regarded as
having a legitimate influence upon it:

> The Crown Prosecution Service acts in the public interest, not just in the
> interests of any one individual. But Crown prosecutors must always think
> very carefully about the interests of the victim, which are an important
> factor, when deciding where the public interest lies.
>
> (Code for Crown Prosecutors, appended to
> CPS Annual Report 1993–4, London: HMSO)

3   That is to say, a negotiation between prosecution and defence with the
object (for the prosecution) of obtaining a guaranteed conviction at reduced
cost; (for the court) of saving judicial time; and (for the defendant) of
securing a lesser sentence. The definitive account of this process is still that
of Baldwin and McConville (1977).
4   Royal Commission, 8.36–45
5   Code for Crown Prosecutors, para. 9.1.
6   Letter to *The Times*, 12 January 1993.
7   This was the acquittal rate for Crown Court trials in 1991 (Criminal
Statistics for England and Wales, 1991, HMSO).
8   The Royal Commission on Criminal Justice (8.47) claims to have been told
by the CPS that it is their policy to intervene when the defence 'depart from
the facts in a material aspect' in the course of mitigation.
9   The Royal Commission (*ibid.*) recommended that 'a power be vested in the
judge to prohibit in the last resort the reporting of unsupported allegations
made during a speech in mitigation'.
10   The Victim/Witness in Court schemes (Rock 1993: 331ff) are designed to
combat problems of isolation and intimidation of victims. There was no
such scheme operating in Bristol Crown Court at the time of our research.
11   The Royal Commission recommends that judges 'should be particularly
vigilant to check unfair and intimidatory cross-examination by counsel of
witnesses who in the nature of the case are likely to be distressed and
vulnerable' (8.43).
12   The Commission recommended that the Victim-Witness in Court Scheme
run by Victim Support be extended to all Crown Courts.
13   For example, 'Terror lurks in the witness box', *Observer*, 21 March 1993;
'Trials collapse as fear silences witnesses', *The Sunday Times*, 3 April
1994; Mr Justice Potter, presiding judge on the Northern Circuit, quoted in
The Times, 23 August 1993:

> Witnesses, particularly those who live in areas of high criminal activity
> who may have witnessed crimes and given statements to the police, are,
> when faced with giving evidence in court, either finding they really can't
> recollect what they'd previously vividly recollected or alternatively re-
> fuse to answer on the grounds that they have been intimidated.

14 Miers (1992) considers the question of victim participation in criminal justice decisions and concludes that while victims' preferences should be noted wherever possible, the desirability of going beyond that is not proven. He identifies the difficulties which would attach to going further as:

> the disclosure of confidential information, the right to be represented at least in the forensic setting, the competing process values enshrined in the rules of criminal procedure, the nature of the public interest in prosecution and sentencing, the credibility of and weight to be attached to the victim's preferences, the means by which any duty to consider these preferences is to be enforced by the victim and . . . the cost to the system.

15 See Zedner (1994: 1233–4) for a brief summary of the arguments for and against allowing victims increased influence over prosecutorial discretion.
16 Criminal Justice Act 1988, s. 104.
17 Criminal Justice Act 1982, s. 67.
18 Other evidence (Hough and Mayhew 1983: 28; Maguire 1982: 138–52) indicates that while some victims may have a generalised preference for tough sentences, their views as to what should happen to the offender in their own case may appear lenient in comparison.

8 ASSAULT, PROSECUTION AND THE VICTIM

1 Following the scheme's introduction in 1964 the number of applications rose each year to 1989/90. The 31,590 awards actually made in 1990/91 was a 25 per cent increase on 1989/90. The CICB is encumbered with such a backlog of cases that over 73 per cent of claims take more than 12 months to process (CICB 26th Report, 1990, Cm. 1365, paras 1.2–1.11).
2 Braithwaite and Pettit acknowledge (p. 113) that 'proactive policing' is required if certain crimes are to be 'brought within the reach of effective enforcement', although it transpires that they are referring here to fraud and other 'white collar' crime, rather than to assault.

Bibliography

Arnold, T.W. (1969) 'Law as symbolism', in V. Aubert (ed.) *Sociology of Law*, London: Penguin.

Ashworth, A. (1986) 'Punishment and compensation: victims, offenders and the state', *Oxford Journal of Legal Studies* 6: 86–122.

Ashworth, A. (1991) *Principles of Criminal Law*, Oxford: Clarendon Press.

Ashworth, A. (1993) 'Victim impact statements and sentencing', *Criminal Law Review*, July.

Austin, J. (1861) *Lectures on Jurisprudence, Vol. II*, London: Sherratt and Hughes.

Avon & Somerset Constabulary (1991) *Violence in the Home: Can We Help?*.

Baldwin, J. and McConville, M. (1977) *Negotiated Justice*, Oxford: Martin Robertson.

Barron, J. (1990) *Not Worth the Paper . . .?*, Bristol: Women's Aid Federation.

Beattie, J.M. (1986) *Crime and the Courts in England, 1660–1800*, Oxford: Clarendon Press.

Berger, P.L. and Luckmann, T. (1966) *The Social Construction of Reality: a treatise in the sociology of knowledge*, London: Allen Lane, Penguin Press.

Biderman, A.D. (1966) 'Social indicators and goals', in R.A. Bauer (ed.) *Social Indicators*, Cambridge, Mass.: The MIT Press.

Blackstone, Sir William (1778) *Commentaries on the Laws of England* [Selections, Edited, with an introduction by Gareth Jones (1979), London: Macmillan].

Blair, I. (1985) *Investigating Rape*, London: Croom Helm.

Blumberg, A. (1969) 'The practice of law as confidence game', in V. Aubert (ed.) *Sociology of Law*, London: Penguin.

Board of Visitors, HMP Wandsworth (1992) *Annual Report*.

Bottomley, A. and Coleman, C. (1976) 'Criminal statistics: the police role in the discovery and detection of crime', *International Journal of Criminology and Penology* 4: 33.

Bottomley, A.K. and Coleman, A.C. (1980) 'Police effectiveness and the public: the limitations of official crime rates', in R.V.G. Clarke and J.M. Hough (eds) *The Effectiveness of Policing*, Aldershot: Gower.

Bottoms, A.E. and McClean, J.D. (1976) *Defendants in the Criminal Process*, London: Routledge and Kegan Paul.

Boyle, C. (1993) 'Guilt, innocence, and truth', *Criminal Law Forum* 4: 3.

Braithwaite, J. and Pettit, P. (1990) *Not Just Deserts: Towards a Republican Theory of Punishment*, Oxford: Clarendon Press.

Bussman, K. (1992) 'Morality, symbolism, and criminal law: chances and limits of mediation programmes', in H. Messmer and H.-U. Otto (eds), *Restorative Justice on Trial*, Dordrecht: Kluwer.

Campbell, T. (1984) 'Compensation as punishment', *University of New South Wales Law Journal* 7: 338–61.

Chatterton, M.R. (1983) 'Police work and assault charges', in M. Punch (ed.) *Control in the Police Organisation*, London: MIT Press.

Christie, N. (1977) 'Conflicts as property', *British Journal of Criminology* 17: 1.

Christie, N. (1986a) 'Crime control as drama', *Journal of Law and Society* 13: 1.

Christie, N. (1986b) 'The ideal victim' in E.A. Fattah (ed.) *From Crime Policy to Victim Policy*, London: Macmillan.

Clarkson, C., Cretney, A., Davis, G. and Shepherd, J. (1994) 'Assaults: the relationship between seriousness, criminalisation and punishment', *Criminal Law Review* 57: 1.

Clarkson, C. and Keating, H.M. (1994) *Criminal Law: Text and Materials* (3rd edition), London: Sweet and Maxwell.

Cretney, A., Davis. G., Clarkson, C. and Shepherd, J. (1994) 'Criminalising assault: the failure of the offence against society model', *British Journal of Criminology* 34: 1.

Criminal Injuries Compensation Board (1990) *Report*, Cm. 1365, London: HMSO.

Criminal Statistics for England and Wales (1992), London: HMSO.

Crown Prosecution Service (1994) *CPS Annual Report 1993–4*, London: HMSO.

Cunningham, J. (1990) 'Thieving in the City', *The Guardian*, 20 December 1990.

Cuthbert, M., Lovejoy, F. and Fulde, G. (1991) 'Investigation of the incidence and analysis of cases of alleged violence reporting to St Vincent's Hospital', in D. Chappell, P. Grabowsky and H. Strang (eds) *Australian Violence: contemporary perspectives*, Canberra: Australian Institute of Criminology.

Dahrendorf, R. (1985) *Law and Order*, London: Stevens & Sons.

Davidoff, L. and Dowds, L. (1989) 'Recent trends in crimes of violence against the person in England and Wales', *Research Bulletin No. 27*, London: Home Office Research and Planning Unit.

Davidoff, L. and Greenhorn, M. (1991) 'Violent crime', Paper delivered to the 1991 British Criminology Conference (London: Home Office).

Davis, G. (1992) *Making Amends*, London: Routledge.

Davis, R.C. (1983) 'Victim/witness non-cooperation: a second look at a persistent phenomenon', *Journal of Criminal Justice* 11: 287–99.

Dobash, R.E. and Dobash, R.P. (1991) Paper to the 1991 British Criminology Conference (University of Cardiff).

Duff, R.A. (1990) *Intention, Agency and Criminal Liability*, Oxford: Basil Blackwell.

Edwards, S. and Halpern, A. (1992) 'The progress towards protection', *New Law Journal* 142: 798–800.

Faragher, T. (1985) 'The police response to violence against women in the home', in J. Pahl (ed.) *Private Violence and Public Policy*, London: Routledge.

Fattah, E.A. (ed.) (1986) *From Crime Policy to Victim Policy*, London: Macmillan.

Feinberg, J. (1984) *Harm to Others*, New York: Oxford University Press.

Fiss, O.M. (1984) 'Against settlement', *Yale Law Journal* 93.

Friedman, L.N. (1975) *The Legal System*, New York: Russell Sage Foundation.

Garland, D. (1990) *Punishment and Modern Society*, Oxford: Clarendon Press.

Garofalo, J. (1977) *The Police and Public Opinion*, Washington, D.C.: National Criminal Justice Information and Statistics Service.

Genn, H. (1988) 'Multiple victimisation', in M. Maguire and J. Pointing (eds) *Victims of Crime: A New Deal?*, Milton Keynes: Open University Press.

Goldstein, A. (1982) 'Defining the role of the victim in the criminal prosecution', *Mississippi Law Journal*, 52: 515–61.

Gottfredson, G.D. (1989) 'The experiences of serious and violent victimisation', *Pathways to Criminal Violence*, California: Sage.

Gottfredson, M.R. (1981) 'On the etiology of criminal victimisation', *Journal of Criminal Law and Criminology* 72: 714–26.

Gottfredson, M.R. (1984) *Victims of Crime: The Dimensions of Risk*, Home Office Research Study No. 81, London: HMSO.

Gottfredson, M.R. and Gottfredson, D.M. (1989) *Decision Making in Criminal Justice: Toward the Rational Exercise of Discretion*, New York: Plenum Press.

Gottfredson, M.R. and Hindelang, M.J. (1979) 'A study of the behaviour of law', *American Sociological Review* 44: 1.

Gustafson, R. and Kallinen, H. (1989) 'Changes in the psychological defence system as a function of alcohol intoxication in men', *British Journal of Addiction* 84: 1515–21.

Heaton-Armstrong, A. and Wolchover, D. (1992) 'Recording witness statements', *Criminal Law Review* 55: 3.

Hindelang, M.J., Dunn, C.S., Sutton, L.P. and Aumick, A.L. (1975) *Sourcebook of Criminal Justice Statistics, 1974*, Washington, D.C.: US Government Printing Office.

Hindelang, M.J. and Gottfredson, M.R. (1976) 'The victim's decision not to invoke the criminal justice process' in W. McDonald (ed.) *Criminal Justice and the Victim*, Beverley Hills: Sage.

Hindelang, M.J., Gottfredson, M.R. and Garofalo, J. (1978) *Victims of Personal Crime: An Empirical Foundation for a Theory of Personal Victimisation*, Cambridge, Mass.: Ballinger.

Hodge, J. (1993) 'Alcohol and violence', in P. Taylor (ed.) *Violence in Society*, London: Royal College of Physicians.

Home Office (1990) *Victim's Charter: A Statement of the Rights of Victims*, London: HMSO.

Home Office (1993) *Digest 2: Information on the Criminal Justice System in England and Wales*, London: HMSO.

Home Office (1994) *Social Trends 24*, London: HMSO.

Hood, R. and Sparks, R.F. (1970) *Key Issues in Criminology*, London: Weidenfeld and Nicolson.

Hough, M. (1991) 'Victims of violent crime: findings from the British Crime Survey', Paper to the 1991 British Criminology Conference (London: Home Office).

Hough, M. and Mayhew, P. (1983) *The British Crime Survey: First Report*, Home Office Research Study No. 76, London: HMSO.

Hough, M. and Mayhew, P. (1985) *Taking Account of Crime: Key Findings from the 1984 British Crime Survey*, Home Office Research Study No. 85, London: HMSO.

Hough, M. and Moxon, D. (1985) 'Dealing with offenders: popular opinion and the views of victims', *The Howard Journal* 24: 3.

House of Commons (1993) *Memorandum of Evidence to Home Affairs Select Committee on Domestic Violence*, London: HMSO.

Kelly, Deborah (1990) 'Victim participation in the criminal justice system', in A.J. Lurigio, W.G. Skogan and R.C. Davis (eds) *Victims of Crime: Problems, Policies, and Programs*, Newbury Park, CA: Sage.

Kemp, C, Norris, C. and Fielding, N.G. (1992) *Negotiating Nothing: Police Decision-Making in Disputes*, London: Avebury.

Law Commission (1992) *Domestic Violence and Occupation of the Family Home*, Law Commission Report No. 207, London: HMSO.

Law Commission (1994) *Binding Over*, Law Commission Report No. 222, London: HMSO.

Levi, M. (1994) 'Violent crime', in M. Maguire, R. Morgan and R. Reiner (eds) *The Oxford Handbook of Criminology*, Oxford: Oxford University Press.

Lurigio, A.J., Skogan, W.G. and Davis, R.C. (eds) (1990) *Victims of Crime: Problems, Policies, and Programs*, Newbury Park, CA: Sage.

McCabe, S. and Sutcliffe, F. (1978) *Defining Crime*, Oxford: Basil Blackwell.

McConville, M, Sanders, A. and Leng, R. (1991) *The Case for the Prosecution*, London: Routledge.

McDonald, W.F. (1976) *Criminal Justice and the Victim*, Beverley Hills: Sage.

McHugh, M. and Thompson, C (1991) 'The role of alcohol in the commission of crimes of violence', Paper to the 1991 British Criminology Conference.

Maguire, M. (1982) *Burglary in a Dwelling*, London: Heinemann Educational.

Maguire, M. and Corbett, C. (1987) *The Effects of Crime and the Work of Victim Support Schemes*, Aldershot: Gower.

Mawby, R. (1988) 'Age, vulnerability and the impact of crime', in M. Maguire and J. Pointing (eds) *Victims of Crime: A New Deal?*, Milton Keynes: Open University Press.

Mayhew, P. (1984) 'The effects of crime: victims, the public and fear', Council of Europe, 16th Criminological Research Conference, Strasburg.

Mayhew, P. (1991) 'A perspective on victimization rates from the 1989 International Crime Survey', Paper to the 1991 British Criminology Conference.

Mayhew, P, Elliott, D. and Dowds, L. (1989) *The 1988 British Crime Survey*, Home Office Research Study No. 111, London: HMSO.

Mayhew, P., Aye Maung, N. and Mirrlees-Black, C. (1993) *The 1992 British Crime Survey*, Home Office Research Study No. 132, London: HMSO.

Miers, D. (1976) 'Victims of crime: sources of financial redress', *Home Office Research Bulletin*, No. 3, London: Home Office.

Miers, D. (1978) *Responses to Victimisation*, Abingdon: Professional Books.

Miers, D. (1992) 'The responsibilities and the rights of victims of crime', *Modern Law Review* 55: 4.

Mills, C. Wright (1959) *The Sociological Imagination*, New York: Oxford University Press.

Moonman, J. (1987) 'Violence in the Home' in J. Moonman (ed.) *Violence in the Home*, London: Frank Cass.

Morley, R. and Mullender, A. (1992) 'Hype or hope? The importation of pro-arrest policies and batterers' programmes from North America to Britain as key measures for preventing violence against women in the home', *International Journal of Law and the Family* 6: 265–88.

O'Brien, E. (1986) *Asking the Victim: A Study of the Attitudes of Some Victims of Crime to Reparation and the Criminal Justice System*, Gloucestershire Probation Service.

Pannick, D. (1987) *Judges*, Oxford: Oxford University Press.

Pease, K. (1988) *Judgements of Crime Seriousness: Evidence from the British Crime Survey 1984*, Research and Planning Unit Paper 44, London: HMSO.

Phillips, S. and Cochrane, R. (1991) 'Assaults against the police: three studies conducted in the Midlands', in A.K. Bottomley, T. Fowles and R. Reiner (eds) *Criminal Justice: Theory and Practice*, London: British Society of Criminology.

Raine, J. and Smith, R (1991) *The Victim/Witness in Court Project; Report of the Research Programme*, London: Victim Support.

Reiner, R. (1985) *The Politics of the Police*, London: Harvester.

Roberts, P. and Willmore, C. (1993) *The Role of Forensic Science Evidence in Criminal Proceedings*, Submission to the Royal Commission on Criminal Justice, Research Study No. 11, London: HMSO.

Rock, P. (1990) *Helping Victims of Crime: the Home Office and the Rise of Victim Support in England and Wales*, Oxford: Clarendon Press.

Rock, P. (1993) *The Social World of an English Crown Court*, Oxford: Clarendon Press.

Royal Commission on Criminal Justice (1993), Cm. 2263, London: HMSO.

Sanders, A. (1988) 'Personal violence and public order', *International Journal of the Sociology of Law* 16: 359.

Schneider, A.L. (1976) 'Victimization surveys and criminal justice system evaluation', in W.G. Skogan (ed.) *Sample Surveys of the Victims of Crime*, Cambridge, Mass.: Ballinger.

Sellin, T. and Wolfgang, M. (1964) *The Measurement of Delinquency*, New York: Wiley.

Shah, R. and Pease, K. (1992) 'Crime, race and reporting to the police', *Howard Journal* 31: 3.

Shapland, J. (1984) 'Victims, the criminal justice system and compensation', *British Journal of Criminology* 24: 2.

Shapland, J. (1986) 'Victim assistance and the criminal justice system', in E.A. Fattah (ed.) *From Crime Policy to Victim Policy*, London: Macmillan, pp. 118–236.

Shapland, J., Willmore, J. and Duff, P. (1985) *Victims in the Criminal Justice System*, Aldershot: Gower.

Shapland, J. and Cohen, P. (1987) 'Facilities for victims: the role of the police and the courts', *Criminal Law Review*, January.

Shepherd, J., Pearce, N.X., Scully, C. and Leslie, I.J. (1987) 'Rates of violent crime from hospital records', *Lancet* 8573: 1473–81.

Shepherd, J., Shapland, M. and Scully, C. (1989) 'Recording by the police of violent offences: an accident and emergency department perspective', *Medicine, Science and the Law* 29: 3.

Shepherd, J., Robinson, L. and Levers, B. (1990a) 'Roots of urban violence', *Injury* 21: 139–141.

Shepherd, J., Qureshi, R., Preston, M.S. and Levers, B.G.H. (1990b) 'Psychological distress after assaults and accidents', *British Medical Journal*, 13 October.

Shepherd, J., Shapland, M., Pearce, N. and Scully, C. (1990c) 'Pattern, severity and aetiology of injuries in victims of assault', *Journal of the Royal Society of Medicine* 83.

Shepherd, J. (1990a) 'Violent crime in Bristol: an Accident and Emergency Department perspective', *British Journal of Criminology*, 30/3.

Shepherd, J. (1990b) 'Victims of personal violence: the relevance of Symonds' model of psychological response and loss theory', *British Journal of Social Work* 20: 309–32.

Shepherd, J., Ali, M.A., Hughes, A.O. and Levers, B.G.H. (1993) 'Trends in urban violence: a comparison of Accident Department and police records', *Journal of the Royal Society of Medicine* 86: 87–9.

Sheptycki, J. (1992) 'The limitations of the concept of the domestic violence incident in policing and social scientific discourses', in A.K. Bottomley, T. Fowles and R. Reiner (eds) *Criminal Justice: Theory and Practice*, London: British Society of Criminology.

Smith, D.J. and Gray, J. (1983) 'The police in action', *Police and People in London*, vol. IV, London: PSI.

Smith, L. (1989) *Domestic Violence: An Overview of the Literature*, London: HMSO.

Straus, M.A., Gelles, R.J. and Steinmetz, K. (1980) *Behind Closed Doors: Violence in the American Family*, Newbury Park, CA: Sage.

Sparks, R.F., Genn, H.G. and Dodd, D.J. (1977) *Surveying Victims*, London: Wiley.

Teubner, G. and Wilke, H. (1984) Kontext und Autonomie: Gesellschaftliche Selbsteuerung durch reflexives Recht, *Zeitschrift für Rechtssoziologie* 5: 4–35.

Tomsen, S., Homel, R. and Thommeny, J. (1991) 'The causes of public violence: situational and other factors', in D. Chappell, P. Grabosky and H. Strang (eds) *Australian Violence: Contemporary Perspectives*, Canberra: Australian Institute of Criminology.

Victim Support (1992) *Domestic Violence: Report of a National Inter-Agency Working Party*, London: Victim Support.

Von Hirsch, A. (1985) *Past or Future Crimes: Deservedness and Dangerousness in the Sentencing of Criminals*, Manchester: Manchester University Press.

Von Hirsch, A. and Jareborg, N. (1991) 'Gauging criminal harm', *Oxford Journal of Legal Studies* 11.

Walmsley, R. (1986) *Personal Violence*, Home Office Research Study No. 89, London: HMSO.

Weisstub, D.N. (1986) 'Victims of crime in the criminal justice system', in E. Fattah (ed.) *From Crime Policy to Victim Policy*, London: Macmillan.

Williams, K.M. (1976) 'The effects of victim characteristics in the disposition of violent crimes', in W. McDonald (ed.) *Criminal Justice and the Victim*, Beverley Hills: Sage.

Wolfgang, M. (1958) *Patterns of Criminal Homicide*, New York: Wiley.
Yarsuvat, D. (1989) 'Criminal policy regarding protection of the victim', in E. Viano (ed.) *Crime and its Victims*, New York: Hemisphere.
Zedner, L. (1994) 'Victims', in M. Maguire, R. Morgan and R. Reiner (eds) *The Oxford Handbook of Criminology*, Oxford: Oxford University Press.
Ziegenhagen, E. (1978) *Victims, Crime and Social Control*, New York: Praeger.

Index